THE POSITIVE OF MY TRIPLE-NEGATIVE BREAST CANCER

Pearls of Wisdom from the Patient's Perspective

Tricia J. Griffith

ISBN: 979-8-9878555-4-6

DEDICATION

This book is dedicated to Breast Cancer Thrivers determining their next steps. Remember to give yourself grace for the step you are currently on.

I also dedicate it to those who gave me grace as I walked along this path and held me when I stumbled.

CONTENTS

ACKNOWLEDGMENTS

To my family, friends, First Baptist Church members, West Coast Prayer Call Warriors, Chapter Sorors (especially 94++), sorority sisters near and far, and Momentum Education facilitators and coaches... THANK YOU all for participating in my journey then and now.

Special thanks to my Mother, Eldria, who was a pillar of strength for me throughout my journey. And my brother Kerry, sister Loretta, and friend Donna who were at almost every appointment for the duration of a year. My nephews, for the laughter is medicine support during the 3118 House on the Hill get-well retreats. And Adrienne and Rashida for hours of critical phone support.

A host of people in my circle were there praying for me, taking me to appointments when asked, and giving advice, solicited or not. I treasure you all, and I thank you!

This was a pivotal point in my life, and I sustained it due to those around me. It wasn't the best of times, but it wasn't the absolute worst. It was hard, but I am better for it, still living life, and I look forward to many more good times because of what you all have done for me and with me.

And to my Dear Lord and Savior that saw it fit to see me through the darkest of days. I would be nowhere without my faith in God. Thank you, Father, for your grace, mercy, and love.

PREFACE

There is life during and after breast cancer.

I realize that's not the message we've been conditioned to believe, but trust me–it's true. The journey is hard at times but bearable. Even in the darkest hours, it can often produce hope, joy, and laughter...if you so choose. It may sound simple; however, it's an important choice that has to be made.

The first and most important key I've found to be true throughout surviving this journey is the power of *choice*. We have all heard sayings like, *"Turn your gray skies blue," "Turn your frown into a smile,"* or *"Fake it until you make it."* These are more than clichés–they are a mindset. To experience joy, we must intentionally choose joy!

This is my personal journey–how I navigated the path from darkness to brighter days. I'm ready to share what tragedy taught me and what triumph brought me. As well as money-saving tips and how to tap into resources you may not realize are available to you. By sharing my story as a breast cancer survivor, I hope to inspire you to move forward fearlessly!

But, before we begin…

The contents of this book are not meant to diagnose, treat, or cure you. This is simply my side of the journey. How I've used the advice that I received from doctors, my circle of family, friends, and other survivors to thrive. I'm sharing what I did to make it, so you can, too. Everything between these pages rings true for me, but please be warned that you *must* discuss what's best for you with your doctor and medical team.

Statistically, more people are living after being diagnosed with cancer rather than dying from it. You have the best chance on Earth to live a happy, healthy, long life as long as you listen to your body and the medical professionals assigned to you. Additionally, the path I chose with one doctor or center versus another is not to say they were bad choices; they just weren't right for me. For this reason, some names of people and places depicted in this book have been changed.

Finally, I should warn you that some parts of this book may be triggering. But overall, I hope it provides a relatable testimony, sound advice, and more than anything, gives you hope.

LIVING POSITIVELY WITH TRIPLE-NEGATIVE BREAST CANCER

I am Tricia Griffith, and I was diagnosed with Stage 1 Triple-Negative Invasive Ductal Carcinoma, an aggressive form of breast cancer most commonly found in African-American women. Throughout the course of my treatment, I had two breast surgeries, chemotherapy, and radiation. Everyone's journey with cancer will undoubtedly be different; however, we are still a community of survivors, trying our best to make it through.

Some say knowing that you have cancer is the worst feeling in the world, but I believe it's the initial shock that wipes the spirit out of most people. You do not know what's ahead of you or if the harsh treatments you're subjected to will work. Having to brave every day, uncertain, unsure, and unprepared. Some go through the journey alone–others have a village. It can all be overwhelming.

No one wants cancer. I don't wish it on my worst enemy, but getting cancer changed my life forever and for the better. After six years, I feel healthier than ever, living what I consider my best life. I'm even more grounded. There's something about enduring a serious, life-threatening illness that helps you find the strength to take on the worst of times, no matter what they are. I am here to help you along the journey. As a survivor, I can share how I reacted to the world, how the world reacted towards me, and how I wish some reactions would have actually gone.

Remember–everyone's journey is different.

When I was diagnosed, there was no how-to guide to walk me through being an African-American woman faced with fighting cancer in the prime of her life. Yes, we have the internet, and it's vast. However, back then, it wasn't filled with the useful information I was seeking. The niche market on the trials, tribulations, and triumphs of African-Americans fighting breast cancer was left to be desired.

I want to reiterate here that many more people are living with cancer than dying from it. Survivorship and overcoming cancer is ticking upward. I want to help you be a survivor by giving you hope and providing some facts and resources. Even caregivers will gain knowledge on their end as well.

The journey requires plenty of heart work. Read that again because you might have read that sentence, and the brain inserted *HARD* work, and that's okay. Getting back to your healthy self will be HARD work, but the heart work comes with the fight, too. Remaining your most true, authentic self is **heart work**. I can give you all the tips, but in the end, living, surviving, and thriving is up to you and what you choose to do with the information provided. The goal during your cancer journey is to heal and make it through. I decided to write my journey because it helped me to heal, and I want to help others. I have found that sharing your journey helps you heal while helping others heal. They say as you learn, you should teach while continuing to learn.

As I write and remember the lessons I've learned, despite the pain of reliving it, it's still healing for me. There are times when I think, *Wow, this really happened to me*. I sit thinking about why, then pledge to do better, implementing what I've learned to avoid those costly missteps in life that initially led me here. But as I teach, there are lessons that I need to keep learning, too. My sincere hope is that you get it on your first pass.

Cancer isn't easy, but for me, it was needed. I was going down a path where I wasn't happy. I didn't enjoy my work, my romantic relationship wasn't solid, and I wasn't asking for what I truly wanted and needed. Now don't get me wrong—I spoke up and advocated for myself, but it seemingly wasn't enough. I was being, acting, and accepting mediocrity, agreeing to things just to be counted and not miss out. (That's FOMO: *Fear of Missing Out*).

These days, life looks different for me. I treasure every day that I'm alive and see life as a precious gift. The many sleepless nights I endured motivated me to put pen to paper; I wanted to do more for my community, which inspired the birth of this book. Our bodies are consistently speaking, telling us where to go and what to do. I was out doing the work of everyone else, giving my *"yes"* to friends and family, went through a pandemic (still prevalent at the time of this writing), and never stopped to get this done. During my journey, however, I've learned it's okay to say no, and just be. Going through treatment meant spending many days with nothing to do except *be*; at the start of writing this book in 2021, I realized just *being* is just fine. Other's measure of success should not be to the detriment of me.

This book is a positive guide for the person who wants and chooses to live! I talk about my journey and what I (as well as others interviewed) did to make it through. I give suggestions and advice; however, you must do what's best for you with the guidance of a medical professional. Your doctors are the ones whom you have a rapport with and know your situation. Not the infomercial doctor that doesn't know you personally and you can't speak to for a full assessment of your specific condition.

Now that we're clear on that, let's get into these pearls.

Pearl of Wisdom #1: The power of choice is the most important key to surviving this journey.

Pearl of Wisdom #2: Share your journey in a way you're comfortable with, whether big or small. Sharing doesn't mean putting it in a book for the world to see. You may want to have an intimate chat with a small group of family and friends, your therapist, or even write in your journal. Just know that holding it in could be detrimental to your well-being.

Pearl of Wisdom #3: Identify your *why* in everything you do. Why you wake up, why you write, why you're saying yes, why you're saying no. It's more than the reason why; it's the meaning behind what you are doing. It's about a life of purpose.

Pearl of Wisdom #4: Use discernment. During the cancer journey, it may be hard to follow your North Star and stay true to yourself. You're getting solicited and unsolicited advice from everyone, so discernment is key to deciphering what you actually need. I always say take what you need and leave what you don't.

THE HOUSE ON THE HILL

~~~

Growing up in Queens, I was always surrounded by people and love. My childhood home was affectionately known as *3118 - The House on the Hill*. It was the epicenter of the neighborhood, where everything started and ended. This was where all the action was, even for those who didn't live there. Although my fondest memory of my childhood is dancing and singing in our Manhattan apartment surrounded by my mother, father, and sisters, I'll never forget the house in Queens. And everything it stood for–family, belonging, and strength.

I remember doing crossword puzzles and watching *Jeopardy, Family Feud* and *People's Court* with my grandmother. And oh, how I loved cooking with my Aunt Dewdrop and playing double-dutch in the street with my cousins. Then we'd sit on the stoop, watching my brother and older cousin strategize how many cars to take to the beach the next day.

I can't forget the block parties, cookouts, proms, graduations, birthdays, shooting pool in the basement, and the pigeons and the pigeon coup in the back (my uncle used to race pigeons). *3118* was there through thick and thin–marriages, births, divorce, and deaths. And eventually, *3118* witnessed the windstorm of cancer and its treatments. Over five generations of family activities occurred in that house in Queens, and I'm grateful to have experienced them all.

My room was on the second floor of the house. When I couldn't go outside, I remember getting intoxicated off peach Schnapps, then screaming out the window to my boyfriend, slightly older than I was, who stayed out later than me. My room had a terrific front view, but so did my grandmother's room. Lord, did I become her long before I even knew I'd turned into her. Window wide open, poking my head out with no shame. Not even trying to peek as I took in the action outside.

When I hit 32 and moved out of The House on the Hill in favor of a small apartment in the Bronx, my tiny place became ground zero for my friends. Every weekend, my sofa was packed with folks sleeping over, and I even placed a queen-sized air mattress in the living room where they could rest for the night. Living on my own was fun, but my mind constantly raced back to the house in Queens and all the secrets it kept. Like when my cousin and I snuck boys through the front door, who ended up having to jump out the window before my grandmother could climb the steps.

Quite a few family members have lived in the Queens house, using it as a refuge. Some of them left raging mad, but they always returned. I recall the blackout in August of 2003. With no electricity in the house, a bunch of the family hung out half the night on the stoop. It was hot, but fun just shooting the shit.

In 2016, I turned 40 and fell ill. It came as a shock to me because that March I brought in my 40th year of life in beautiful Barbados and then traveled to Paris that July to continue the celebration. But in October, my life changed forever when I was diagnosed with breast cancer.

Naturally, the Queens house once again became ground zero, my point of retreat. One day while lying in my mother's bed, I told her I was sick. My mother had no clue about the test I was taking.

"Mom, I have something to tell you," I said.

"Is it cancer?" she asked without looking at me.

The answer, seemingly lodged in my throat, finally came out. "Yes, Mom. It is."

Just like the main cheerleader in my life that she is and has always been, my mother said, "We are going to beat this thing!"

Shortly after, I chose a treatment center, and *3118* became the focal point of *Operation Get Better*. So as you see, I was a simple girl from simple means, living a pretty simple life. A life I loved without extravagance. I work, I'm a part of a sorority, and I have plenty of family supporting and surrounding me.

GOING BACK HOME

On chemotherapy days, I came home to Queens to convalesce. During this time, my brother had taken over and stopped the house from being a merry-go-round for relatives. The house of happy chaos had finally emptied and was quieter.

The block had changed drastically as well. It was no longer predominately Black, and I didn't know every neighbor on the block. It was a strange feeling, considering that growing up, we knew everyone, and everyone knew us. You couldn't turn on the fire hydrant and leave it running, as everyone had to agree on everything that would happen on the block—even if it was all in fun. It was all about respecting our neighbors. But now, we were fighting loud, obnoxious neighbors who partied too much and for too long without inviting you...even though their guests parked in your driveway! The block had become annoying. Never anywhere to park, but *3118* was still there, and it was still home base.

I was lucky enough to have my mother, brother, and nephews at the house waiting on me hand and foot during this time. I wanted for nothing! I usually visited *Cancer Treatment Centers of America (CTCA)* from Wednesday to Friday, leaving Philadelphia on Saturday morning after a good night's rest. I took off those three days, but after a while, I was able to get down to two days. I thought about the days when I'd only have to visit CTCA for a day, which never came to fruition, as they eventually closed.

Whenever I returned from most of my CTCA trips, my mother had fresh bedding and everything ready for me to relax. I appreciated her so much for that. I slept well, right there in my childhood bedroom. One thing that bothered me was the sheer curtains that were hung in the room. I hated them! But I eventually came to realize that I was allowing my body to wake with the natural circadian cycles. I was up super early with the sun, daydreaming and taking the prayer call under the covers. Sometimes, my eyes welled up with tears as I thought about what I was facing at the moment and what was next.

Eventually, I got up to eat, watch *The View*, watch movies, then take a nap. When my nephews and brother came home from work at different times throughout the day, I'd liven up from being bored out of my mind. By the following Monday or Tuesday, I felt so much better and was ready to work. While work usually drove me a little nutty, focusing on something other than having cancer literally kept me grounded and sane.

While it was imperative for me to rest during chemotherapy, it was also important for me to remain active and keep moving. For me, movement is life! I had to figure out what felt good and what didn't. My doctor advised me not to do anything that hurt or my body didn't agree with. It was the simple things that counted towards my recovery.

The chemotherapy sessions began in February. I wasn't outside too often, so I traipsed up and down the staircase in the house when I had the strength. I made it a point to physically get out of bed every day, go to work, and entertain distant family and friends who visited. It was a relaxing, refreshing time for me. I left one oasis (CTCA) and retreated to Mom's house, still in nirvana, surrounded by love.

Pearl of Wisdom #5: Your physical space may look different, and different people may be around you, but take the love that people extend to you at this time. Try to be "present" as best you can to receive the support that comes your way. Do not try to be everything for everyone. For example, if you are a mother, there are times when you may not feel like cooking for your children or cleaning. There is support for you! I've found a service that will bring cooked meals to you, as well as a low-cost cleaning service to help clean up those messes (refer to the *Appendix* at the end of this book). And by all means, when people ask what they can do for you, tell them!

DR. FABULOUS

~~~

What is therapy to me? Therapy is speaking to someone who listens to you, allows you to talk and get everything out you need to release, and provides feedback and directions on next steps to help you.

I'd been seeing my gynecologist–we'll call her "Dr. Fabulous", since being recommended by my sorority sister, Dr. JCR. I'm not sure how I got so lucky, but sitting in the room with Dr. Fabulous was like therapy to me. My 15-minute sessions usually ended up being 20-30 minutes but felt like an hour of real talk. After our sessions, I always came out feeling better about myself and my life. Talking to her reassured me that everything would either be okay, or she'd detail the steps I needed to get there. Don't get me wrong, I had similar interactions with a lot of my doctors; I seemed to have the luck of the Irish when it came to good doctors, even before cancer came.

Dr. Fabulous was Caucasian, loud, boisterous, and loved to talk! Sitting in the room waiting for her to come in for our appointments, I'd laugh as I heard her vibrant voice speaking to other patients through the center's hallowed walls.

My gynecological issues were multiple and varied. It wasn't until I started seeing Dr. Fabulous that things started to get better. I'd been examined by a gamut of medical professionals of almost every race and gender; however, Dr. Fabulous had a special way of helping me understand what was going on with my body.

It all began one day during the fall of 1998 (my final year of college), when I fainted from abdominal pain. Shortly after, I was diagnosed with fibroids and ovarian cysts. Finishing college meant getting the boot from my mother's health insurance; not being as savvy about my health as I am today, I was left to my own devices. I ended up going to a male doctor, who thought it was best to surgically remove the ovarian cysts without explaining to me that they grow back and the surgery could hurt my chances of getting pregnant in the future. Straight out of college, I had no idea that following the decision to have that surgery, my uterine walls became scarred, and salvaging my eggs before chemotherapy was impossible.

Let me explain.

Fallopian tubes are the female reproductive organs that connect the ovaries and the uterus. Every month during ovulation, an egg is carried in the fallopian tubes from an ovary to the uterus. I had ovarian cysts removed, which caused scar tissue and adhesions on the left side. Since having that surgery, doctors always ask me if I had my ovaries removed because they can't see them via sonogram due to the scarring. As a result of the scarring, I was unsuccessful in preserving my eggs.

My sister Kim reminded me about a mutual friend who was a pathologist at *MD Anderson Medical Center*, and I immediately had the specimen from my ovarian surgery sent to her for review. After checking for size, grade, and possible malignancy, all of my tests came back with good results. Along with the good news, the pathologist told me that she would not have removed the cysts, explaining that they grow back. She also mentioned there are natural ways to avoid some of this until we're ready to conceive and take other courses of action. Unbeknownst to me, the damage was already done, and I embarked on a hunt for a new doctor. Being Black wasn't a requirement, but I definitely wanted a female doctor.

Enter Dr. Fabulous.

Dr. Fabulous took the time to talk to me and give me sound advice, such as to stop wearing panty liners and to let my lady parts breathe. And when I was terribly overwhelmed with anxiety and depression, she told me to start talk therapy, not to jump right into taking medication. She also ran blood work for me that my former primary physician refused to because she didn't see the use in it and didn't know how to interpret the results. Now I had my share of phenomenal doctors, but I had some incredibly shady ones, too.

Dr. Fabulous was the right mix of Western and Eastern Medicine. It was like having my own Christiane Northrup (author of *Women's Bodies, Women's Wisdom*). Christiane Northrup is a famous OB-GYN from the northeast who taught women about the mind and body connection. She appeared on Oprah numerous times; like many women back then, I got all my news from Oprah! Anyway, just like Dr. Northrup, Dr. Fabulous explained a lot to me about the mind and body connection, which is conjoined and holistic. Things can happen in our bodies based on how we feel and interact with the world around us.

From helping me diagnose it, Dr. Fabulous was pivotal in my cancer journey. No matter how many questions I had, she and her assistant were diligent in answering me through the office portal. They answered immediately, never making me wait. They were consistent in calling me and scheduling me for tests and appointments and played intricate roles as the start of my healthcare team.

Now that I've given you some of my background, here's how this whole journey actually started.

October 5, 2016.

I went in for my very first mammogram. I'd turned 40 in March but waited to have the test done until Breast Cancer Awareness Month. Well into 17 years as a member of Alpha Kappa Alpha Sorority Incorporated, every October, I ran health fairs, rallying women to get tested. Because of the role I played, it was only appropriate for me to be counted in the number of women who got screened in October, especially with our chapter's efforts to help the Bronx community to rise from being dead last at #62 in health screenings.

Sometimes, I wonder if delaying my test gave the beast time to grow in me. Nonetheless, my results came back negative, which in doctor speak is a positive thing. "The mammogram results were clear," I was told. "See you in one year." I accepted what they said, but it was what they didn't tell me that would later become a problem. I had *dense breast*, medically known as fibro glandular tissue—which I'd later learn was another contributing factor to my diagnosis.

Being that Dr. Fabulous was on top of her game, providing me with the best care, and the fact that medical regulations were changing, Dr. Fabulous requested that I also get a breast ultrasound to investigate the dense breast issue. I want to be clear—dense breasts do not mean *large* breasts. It simply means that the fatty, dense tissue in women's breasts can make abnormalities more difficult to spot on mammograms.

With my storied past and numerous gynecological issues, Dr. Fabulous and I were doing our best to find the source of the abnormal bleeding I'd been experiencing. At my age, it was crucial for her to conduct a thorough work-up and all the baseline tests I needed to identify what was going on. Consequently, she ordered a breast ultrasound, which was performed the morning of Friday, October 21st. Later that day, Dr. Fabulous called me with the results.

"You should get a breast biopsy," she told me. She must've mistook my stunned silence for nonchalance because she quickly followed up with, "Okay, I will get that scheduled for you. How about Monday?"

My mind was boggled. Throat closing in, I squeezed out a timid "Okay," and disconnected the call.

That Monday morning, my sister Loretta accompanied me to my appointment. Tears burned my face; I didn't feel hope…I felt cancer. Although figuratively, something inside of me already knew that I had cancer. The procedure I had was painful, and they left the clips in me. Why would they leave clips in me?

October 25, 2016, I opened up **MYCHART** account on the computer, reading my results before the doctor could tell me anything. I didn't fully know what everything meant on the pathology report, but I knew what *malignant carcinoma* meant. My close friends whom I opened up to, told me not to worry until I spoke to the doctor. I didn't worry, but I knew.

Of course, Dr. Fabulous retrieved the results the same day as I did. "Come to my office," she ominously called and told me. I woke up that Friday morning, prepared to go in and receive my fate. My boyfriend at the time looked at me and suggested, "You should wear pink today."

...and so I did.

Most of us have either read books, watched movies, or listened to someone's account of them first hearing the words, "*You have cancer.*" Followed by the rush of emotions, feeling lonely, empty, and hopeless. When I arrived at her office, Dr. Fabulous was so gracious and caring. I remember how gentle she was. Her voice was as quiet as I'd ever heard it, almost a whisper as she teetered on the brink of tears, like I'd never witnessed during our relationship. She didn't want to tell me; I didn't want to hear it. But I had no choice.

Suddenly, I was faced with a new reality. It was a brutal shock, and a blow to my heart. I'd had a few days to mentally prepare myself, so I wasn't caught off guard. But I was still hurt. I had already agonized over it, so my reaction in Dr. Fabulous' office was different than the days before. Listening to her speak this time, the tears weren't immediate. My mind didn't race, and I didn't black out or feel like my life was over. I mean, I'd gone through the gamut of those emotions already. It dawned on me that I hadn't shared with my mate that I'd read the results.

My emotionless, still response must have made him think I was inhuman.

My ex is a man of few words. Out of all his many good traits, handling basic human emotions wasn't one of them. Throughout our relationship, I often felt he was unaware and emotionless. His blankness caused me to immerse myself in emotional intelligence books, trying to figure him out. Through my readings, I learned he wasn't cold; he lacked emotional intelligence, which didn't make him a bad person—just human. Sitting in Dr. Fabulous' office with me, he showed a completely different side of himself.

After reading the results, Dr. Fabulous gave us a moment to ourselves. For the first time, I saw tears welling in his eyes. My heart burst open for him in a way it had not in the past.

"I'm sorry for crying," he apologized.

"It's okay," I assured him. "I know this is hard on you."

I would never really come to understand my ex's feelings because I'd unfairly shut him out for so long. The last thing I wanted was for him to see me at my weakest, which ultimately became the downfall of our relationship.

I have to stop here to remind you: Please accept help and love when people give it to you. You can't take on cancer alone! Don't be afraid or ashamed to need help or love. This isn't a sign of weakness, but it's a sign of a well-rounded individual.

Pearl of Wisdom # 6: I'd caution you against reading the report days ahead of seeing your doctor. You may want to review it a day or even a few hours before your visit so you can arm yourself with all the questions swirling through your mind. Do not torture yourself waiting for days on edge!

Upon returning to the room, Dr. Fabulous was more composed. Just like the support she consistently was, she began laying out next steps for me. She explained seeing a breast surgeon was next and even took the time to circle things on the results to show them. Then, they could explain the size, grade, and course of action I needed to take to fight it more in-depth. She also gave me the breast surgeon's name at my center and alerted the department that I would be following up next week.

Taking in my surroundings as we walked from the doctor's office, I was reminded that I live in a big city, and it was my right to explore the best options for my care. Before we got back to our car, my best friends and sorority sisters (Donna and Rashida) called my ex. I refused to speak with them, so he filled them in on what was going on, then asked them to pass the information to my other sorority sister and bestie, Adrienne.

My ex was fairly new in his position at his job, so he headed off to work as soon as we got back home. Truthfully, I needed the time alone to adjust. My life was starting to unravel. What did everything mean? What was next? How was my life going to change?

My apartment was already spotless, but I still went to work, cleaning things that didn't need to be cleaned in order to avoid calling and making the appointment with the breast surgeon. Eventually, I made the call. If I didn't want to be in the dark about my own life, I had to get moving. That day, I literally became the CEO of *Tricia, Incorporated*. First, I called Loretta and shared the results of the biopsy with her. She raced all the way from her job in lower Manhattan and stayed with me until Donna made it to the house.

The sun fell, and Donna stayed the night. I laid in the dark sobbing; Donna had been awake praying and hurried to my side as soon as she heard me crying. She hugged the life back into me! The tears raged on for a few more days, then suddenly stopped. I am a Pisces, the water sign. All my life, I have been intuitive, sensitive, and highly emotional, just like the 12th sign. However, I was determined not to go through this whole process wading through tears and appearing weak. My strategy mostly worked, but a huge breakdown nearly tossed the entire idea out the window.

Let's be clear–I am not clairvoyant. I had no idea cancer was living inside of me or that the possibility of it even existed. And I certainly wasn't aware that cancer cells live inside of each of us, and our every-day actions can trigger them to grow. (Not speaking medically here). In the years prior to my diagnosis, I was dealing with a lot of heavy issues. My body was raging against me, and I was in and out of the doctors and my natural practitioner's offices. My relationship was rocky, I'd been assigned two of the worst projects in my life back to back, and I was traveling extensively for work. As much as I loved to travel, I wasn't fully able to care for myself as I should've been. I dare not blame myself, but cancer knocked, and I opened the door.

And here we are.

The next two years of my life were some of the hardest I'd ever experienced. But with my team of doctors, friends, and family by my side, I was filled with love and hope and was ready for what lay ahead. This journey holds no punches, but for many, the dark-ness offers glimmers of hope. Looking back on some of these stories, there have been many tears; however, there are also some hearty laughs that hit my soul just right. Please enjoy and know that you have the power within you to overcome so much! I found the light in my journey; you can find the light, too.

DECIDING WHO TO TELL

As a late Gen Xer, early Millennial who uses Facebook minimally, Instagram generally and understands Twitter and TikTok, I knew that I wanted to share my journey, but wasn't sure how. First, there are levels to sharing both good and bad news. For example, when someone gets married or someone dies, it's jarring for me to see it first on the internet. If you are in my circle, you will undoubtedly hear any news concerning my life directly from me before it hits the internet streets. That's just me. The internet is an attention grabber; it's all about what will garner the most likes or attention. Very early on, Facebook decided against including a dislike button on the platform and has stood by that decision. For me, the jury is still out on whether this is a good thing.

Sharing your story opens you up to questions, opinions, feedback, and criticism, just as this book will. But look at it this way: Sharing frees us in some way and liberates our souls. That's one less burden to cling to.

Keeping secrets is hard to do. Not only does it eat away at you, it's an unnecessary breeding ground for lying and stress, which should be avoided at all costs when you're fighting for your life!

Think carefully about who you want to share this journey with. With the exception of one person in my life, no matter who I intimately shared my diagnosis with, they were tied to me for life. These are the people who are your core; they will have questions and will want to be kept abreast of your progress. I have a huge network of family and friends. At some point, I broke out in hives, having to repeat the same story to so many different people. In hindsight, I should've put it all in a blog, but I didn't. Maybe documenting my struggles and triumphs would've helped when I was unable to find the words to speak. Eventually, on Saturday, November 5th, I summoned my family to a meeting to discuss everything at once. Anyone who missed the meeting was going to have to find out what was going on from someone else because I refused to regurgitate the same information over and over. It was just too much and too emotional.

I held the meeting in the basement of my childhood home, where I carefully explained my diagnosis, staging, and what my initial treatment would look like. I needed support and didn't want to constantly explain why I couldn't go out or didn't want to engage in a particular activity. Ironically, being stricken with cancer gave me the strength to say no, and end the conversation there. Because I didn't have to if I didn't want to.

You may be thinking I hid behind my disease or used the prognosis as an excuse. Now I'm by no means a martyr, but I know that I was giving more of myself to others than I reserved for me. Constantly trying to prove that I was a good worker, volunteer, team player, family member, and friend. Somewhere along the line, I was living for likes. Running on the fuel of a deadly disease, before realizing I've always had the power to say "no," just because I don't want to.

One of the most difficult parts of the meeting was the reaction from my first cousin, who was unable to attend but dialed in. As soon as she heard I had cancer, she burst into tears, sobbing on the line. Lord, that hurt my soul! Telling her was like telling my own mother. The difference was Mom was very brave and didn't cry–at least not in my presence. It physically hurt me to tell her that her young, spry daughter was going to need her to take care of her again. She'd taken care of me my entire life; she wasn't supposed to have to care for me anymore.

There weren't many questions to answer that night, which was a relief. After the tears dried, the mood shifted to celebratory since my diagnosis was caught early enough to fight it. It was time to get to work and beat this thing! As a family, we always say let's not wait until the funerals to show our support; it blessed my soul to be celebrated before I was on a deathbed. That night, we ate, drank, and were merrier than ever before. This wouldn't be the last time we got together, either. We made plans to gather in my basement again before my first surgery.

As the days and weeks passed, I shared more with my professional networks. At the time, I served as the VP of the National Pan-Hellenic Council of New York City and the logistics chairman of PMI's NYC chapter. I was also an active member of my sorority, all while working a full-time job. Eventually, something was going to have to give. And it did. I stepped down from my position at PMI; however, I stayed on at NPHC. Looking back, I probably should have stepped back from that as well. I was present but not fully functional, which hurt my friendship with the president of the organization.

Even though I was having a tough time, I still managed to plan a successful Founders' Day Weekend in 2018 for the NPHC. I continued working full-time and was pretty successful corporately, as well as in the work I did for the sorority. With the approval of my doctors, I continued attending sorority conferences and executing successful events, like the breast cancer walk and breast health information sessions for the sorority and other external organizations.

Pearl of Wisdom #7: (For caretakers, family, and friends): Once you are a part of the coveted circle, there are rules of engagement.

1. You're a *confidant*. This is not your information to re-share unless given permission.

2. You're here to *listen*, not contribute. Don't bring down the patient with your own crying and complaining about the direness of the situation.

I read an article in the LA Times, detailing the *Ring Theory* by Susan Silk and Barry Goldman. In the *Ring Theory*, you draw a number of rings (circles) on a piece of paper. The patient (or person with any issue), is written in the center circle. Next, draw another circle around the first. In that circle, write the name of the person(s) next closest to the patient and the issue at hand. You can keep drawing larger circles and adding names of extended family and friends as needed.

The objective of this exercise is simply to understand that the person in the middle can basically say and do what they want to help them release their emotions, like screaming, *This is unfair!* Or, *Why me?* Let's be clear, everyone has the choice to say and do what they want as well; however, the goal is not to bring those rants to the patient–they already have enough to deal with. You can lament or complain to others in your circle or perhaps those on an outer ring, anyone but the patient.

In my personal opinion, this circle also denotes who you can talk to about the patient's diagnosis. You are not allowed to share with those that were not originally privy to the information from ground zero. This is crucial to the trust and confidence of the person experiencing this ordeal. Telling someone who shouldn't have been told, the patient may shut down, and their trust in you is broken. You will see how the *Ring Theory* plays out during my first treatment.

Circling back to the cousin who was crying during my cancer announcement, I totally understood...her heart hurt for me, but it wasn't helpful at that moment. I couldn't allow myself to get sidetracked; I simply remained calm. As for the patient, your family and friends didn't cause cancer. Don't take out your frustrations on them, and know that you won't be the center of attention forever. Wield your powers wisely, and do not abuse your support system.

If you'd like to try the *Ring Theory*, refer to the *Appendix*.

GET ORGANIZED

~~~

I am a project manager by trade, so every assessment or skill test puts me in an analyzer category. My life has always been detailed and organized, and my *Type A* personality won't allow me to stay in chaos too long.

From the time I was born all the way up until *C-Day*, I've always retained my immunization records, doctor's notes, and medical records. When the time came to fight cancer, I already understood the importance of keeping a book of notes. No matter what doctor I saw or who I talked to, I documented each interaction. In the event I was unable to do it myself, I had the caretaker who accompanied me jot down the details for me. Because of my diligence, I can pinpoint the dates of most events during my cancer journey–who said what, when, and why. Actually, I can do this with almost any event in my life. It may not be on my brain, but I guarantee you it's documented somewhere–usually in my daily planner.

Cancer is a much bigger deal than day-to-day activities, so I repurposed a pink binder I'd been holding onto to meticulously keep track of everything. I still have that book until this day. Appointment days and times, specific doctor's notes, drawings, my feelings on specific days, research, and my results. Everything is in that book. Keeping track of this time in your life is imperative. Some want to memorialize it, others want to quickly get through it. I am a facts girl; I want to get to the why and learn from it. Also, I needed to keep track of the holistic supplements and remedies I was taking, especially regarding how they made me feel. See, most holistic or naturopathic supplements do not have contraindications with big pharma drugs, but it is still important to document what you're putting inside your body. For example, while garlic is good for you, you should stop taking it as a supplement prior to any surgery you may have because garlic thins the blood.

Again, my experience is my own. You'll need to do what's best for you, but I think it's highly important to share what did and did not work for me so you'll have a starting point when connecting with your doctors. And while I'm here, there's something you need to know about your appointments, too.

I learned very quickly that this journey exposes you to the same redundant questions over and over.

- *When did you get this test?*
- *When did your menstruation start/stop?*
- *When is/was your surgery?*

- *When is/was chemo?*

- *When is/was radiation?*

Be ready to have these same questions fired at you by family, friends, doctors, and nurses.

For me, the answers were easy to remember; however, the repetitiveness can easily trigger trauma. I wrote out my responses ahead of time, which you may find helpful, too. One–so you don't get any part of it incorrect, and two–you want to have the answers ready for your doctors. Now if you are over relaying this information, let your caregiver handle it. If you stay within the same network or facility, they can easily look up the information they're asking for. Especially because nurses and doctors are often double-checking what was entered in the system to ensure that the correct person is sitting in front of them. Right now, I know you may feel as though you're their only patient, but understand doctors have so many patients, it's their responsibility to ask questions without assumptions. Keep in mind there are also times when inaccurate notes are entered into the system, so it's best to answer any and all questions asked without pushback.

Because I jumped around quite a bit during my care, I've been through the questions a thousand times more than the average person. There was a nurse at one facility who asked no matter how many times I saw her, "So you never had chemo?" Inside, I was livid! On the exterior, I remained remarkably calm. I mean, could this lady not see my PORT? A port is a small device implanted under your skin (via a quick surgery), and is used to administer medications (like chemotherapy), and can also be used for drawing blood.

I elected to have a port implanted for a better quality of care, especially since I hate needles and was advised my veins could collapse. Opting for the port was the best thing I could do for my comfort. In any event, things like answering the same obvious question multiple times is easily upsetting. In my case, it appeared the nurse just wasn't paying attention. She kept her head down, reading from her notes as opposed to fully interacting with me.

Reputable doctors do their research before entering the room, greet you by name, ask how you're feeling, and sometimes offer you lunch. At least, that was my experience. The facility I went to for most of my journey was so small I could literally be on the line ahead of my doctor and sitting four feet from the doctor in the cafeteria. It's hit or miss whether or not you get an attentive doctor or nurse as it is, so I urge you to give your doctors grace. I truly believe most of them are doing the best they can with the load they have. So please keep that in mind when you're feeling frustrated or impatient.

Prior to having surgery (if one is scheduled for you), your doctor will confirm and reconfirm what they are working on with regard to your case. Also, be prepared for them to write on your skin–this is to be sure they are working on the correct limb. There will be so much coming at you; try as best you can to be organized. Show up to every appointment armed with your facts and data; ask plenty of questions to keep yourself informed. This is your life and your body, and you only get one!

I often flip through my pink binder, reflecting upon my life and feelings during that time. Seeing it in print is a mark of achievement for me. This journey isn't a good time, but it's your *life*. I never want to be forced to repeat lessons that I should've gotten the first time. My binder is like the African Adinkra Symbol Sankofa–Return and get it; understand the concept/message the first time so as to not go through it again. Taking time to reflect upon my journey and my notes helps me never to forget where I came from and where I'm headed to.

Sometimes, the journey is a whirlwind. Other times, it's slow as molasses. Documenting the journey is helpful and allows you to go back to think about those lightning-speed times months or years later. You may recall something you didn't initially catch in the moment. When I receive a request to speak regarding my journey or am asked how a certain drug made me feel, I know I can always pull out my binder, just in case the facts don't come off the top of my head.

Finally, my binder helps me to assist others. The network of survivors share experiences with each other, and I like to come from a factual place, freely giving all the information that I have. I know this may sound weird, but my binder brings me peace and joy. It's one of the main reasons I'm able to write this book today.

A giant binder isn't a requirement–you may prefer a small notebook, and that's okay. I just recommend that you have a secure place to store your medical history. Though similar, this record is different from a journal; however, I treated my binder as one. It only made sense for me to store the facts, doctor's notes, drawings, and my responses together. If a doctor prescribed a particular drug and it ended up making me sick, I needed to have that information at my fingertips. It also helped to see my emotional responses and triggers. Was I scared, tired, happy, or sad? It's all right there for me to see.

I'm not telling you what to do, but I am asking that you please get your affairs in order. Just as we buy insurance for our homes and cars, life insurance and medical insurance for our health, you need to document your will, living will, power of attorney, etc. There's a quote I'm sure we've all heard: *I'm as serious as cancer.* Cancer is serious! We hope for the best but have to prepare for the worst. A part of being organized is preparing for the worst. If you don't already have these items in place, you can work with the medical facility to get it done. When you feel up to it, consider working with a lawyer regarding wills and estate planning. This may seem like a lot on top of caring for your health, but it doesn't have to take long and will protect you and your family. I also recommend survivors and caregivers complete the following:

- Health care proxy
- Last will and testament
- Living will
- Power of attorney
- Appointment of agent to control disposition of remains

Pearl of Wisdom #8: Get organized and get your affairs in order. Create a system that works best for you and will help you better manage this aspect of your life.

JOB

~~~

At the time of my diagnosis, I was working at ADP in insurance benefits. Working in benefit implementation for the majority of my career, I understood packages very well. The funny thing is, I'd never taken the time to read my entire plan and didn't fully comprehend all of the benefits that I had access to.

Most people (myself included) want to make sure that we have benefits in place, especially medical and dental. Vision was the top tier for me since I've been in glasses since 3rd grade. For those who are still in corporate jobs, the most important coverage you'll need is short and long-term disability. I knew I had the coverage but wasn't aware of the specifics. It didn't take long for me to get up to speed on my health plans. At some point along the way, my company even sent me a printed book of over 150 pages with all the benefit details I needed. I read the book cover to cover, as it explained all the benefits that were available to me. It's daunting for some, but I compared it to figuring out what my clients' documents meant and explaining it to my team.

You could say I was fortunate to have discovered I had cancer when I did. By then, both my deductible and out-of-pocket maximum were paid, and my health plan was fully covered at 100%. Outside of knowing your health plans at work, as you would do when facing any critical illness, make it a priority to know your rights as an employee as well as your company's policies.

When the situation is critical, you won't have time to figure it out. Get to know your plan, NOW. Doing it for a living took the stress off me, but it could be daunting for you. A good start would be setting aside time each day to review different parts of your plan until you've navigated all the way through. Emphasis on the short and long-term disability plans. My organization had just instituted a critical care plan; if by chance you contracted cancer or heart disease, they would pay an estimated $30,000 towards our medical expenses. Unfortunately, I fell short on that plan–I was diagnosed in October and the benefits wouldn't kick in until January 1st of the following year.

I hope I never have to experience this again, but I have the right insurance in place now. While all insurance is not the same, the breakdowns are similar. It's like car insurance–you purchase it with the hopes of never having to use it, especially in a fender bender. But you have it in your pocket anyway, just in case. It's the same for medical insurance and life insurance. Know all your plan benefits, just in case.

After my diagnosis, the appointments came so swiftly and furiously, it was nauseating. *And there is something that I want to put out there that may be controversial.* Did you know that you don't have to sneak to your doctor's appointments? That's what sick time is for, as long as you can show documentation and proof of your appointments. See, I used to "sneak" out of work during my lunch break to go to the doctor, not to be secretive, but because I didn't want to use my Paid Time Off (PTO). No one told me seeing my doctor didn't require using PTO–it's considered sick time (again, with proof).

Before I went into remission, there were times when I was secretive. Why? Because I felt like I didn't have to explain why I was going to the doctor, all anyone needed to know was that I was going. I didn't want to share anything with my employer or anyone else until I completely understood what was going on with me. It's important to know the difference and understand your reason why. I don't care if I was going to the podiatrist to get my toenails clipped or going in for breast surgery; I had the final say on what and who I divulged the information to. What you tell your manager is up to you.

To recap, here is an organizational plan for you to follow:

- Read your benefits plan carefully.

- Fill out the necessary paperwork and keep copies of everything.

- Take time off as you need for appointments without stress or fear of retribution and losing your job. You'll only make yourself sicker, panicking over whether you'll be back from your appointment in time for a meeting or something else they want you to do. *Sick time is there for you to use.* I made myself sick, scrambling to and from appointments on extended breaks.

I've always been nervous about losing my job. Every year during a certain time period, there comes a point when the staff is cut, and I didn't want to be on the chopping block. My story began in October; however, it ran into that window when cuts happened, so naturally, I was afraid. Each time I took off, it felt like it could be the end for me, and it shouldn't have been that way. That's a cancerous way of thinking! So, I want you to know right here, right now, that the *Family Medical Leave Act (FMLA)* is in place to protect your job.

Giving your job specific, intimate details isn't necessary; however, it's imperative to formally submit what you can. It's not a complicated process, but it is quite involved. Referring back to what I mentioned earlier, keeping copies of paperwork and information will limit the issues you run into. Make sure you have copies of everything to reproduce when you need to without starting over.

Pearl of Wisdom #9: FMLA protects your job; short and long-term disability protects your salary. States like New York also have added protection under state FMLA Laws.

Enacting FMLA and disability benefits basically involves filling out the paperwork, having your doctors sign it, and then submitting the claim. The tricky part is how much time off you will receive with pay. It's not all difficult; however, it's strict, by the book and letter of the law.

For my first surgery, I wanted more than two weeks off because, as it turns out, this cancer thing was getting in the way of a very important trip. I had surgery on Tuesday, November 29, 2016. From that point, I had two weeks off. But I wanted a month off, as my trip was scheduled for December 14th. My doctor only signed for two weeks, so I came back to work, then turned around and took my trip, using my PTO. In hindsight, I realize you cannot have it both ways. If FMLA is there to support you when you or a loved one is sick, you cannot expect a doctor to extend the time off for a recreational trip.

I still cannot believe that I was able to take the trip. Everything was so close together: surgery, recovery time, follow-up visits for results and to track my progress, making sure I was healing with no infections or unusual swelling, and ensuring I had everything I needed.

I was ecstatic that my doctors cleared me to take a much needed getaway. I barely thought about the risk though. I knew about swelling as I had to keep my super small (but cute) Victoria's Secret compression tops on, but knowing what I know now...I should've been wearing a lymphedema compression arm sleeve too. At the time, I hadn't stopped using that arm for blood pressure checks and to have blood drawn. Here is the issue with that: In my first surgery, I had nodes removed in a procedure called a *Sentinel Lymph Node Biopsy*, which checks to see if the cancer has spread.

Having lymph nodes removed makes you prone to swelling, as there are less avenues for your blood to drain into the rest of your body. For example, I was advised to do my best to shield my right arm from bites because the body sends blood (and other bodily fluids) to the area to heal the wound. After that, the fluids are drained back into your body for homeostasis; however, depending on how many nodes you've had removed, the drainage either takes time or stops and causes Lymphaemda or swelling.

Some doctors advise ceasing drawing blood and taking blood pressure from the arm with the nodes removed. I understood but was unaware that you should also wear a compression sleeve on that arm as needed. This would've been good to know since a little over two weeks post-surgery, I was on a plane, prone to blood clotting and swelling without even knowing it. Today, I never fly without wearing a compression sleeve. At least I know now; God protects fools and babies. Oh, and the germs! I was out of the bandages and healing well, but *what if*. Especially now that we've entered the COVID era. It's scary to even think about.

In the end, I'm not sure how or if you've adequately prepared yourself, family, friends, or your place of employment for this battle, but you *must*. In terms of work, my detail-oriented nature is what helped me. My plans had plans, and my notes had notes! I literally left a breadcrumb trail of documents for my coworkers, which assisted them in helping me. Others were able to pick up the slack while I was out with ease. If I hadn't shared, I wouldn't have been helped; there was no other way. The compassion and care I received from my coworkers and managers was heart-warming–it was a relief knowing they were on my side.

Back then, I had multiple managers, but one, in particular, stood out to me. We lived in different states, never physically met, and had different cultural backgrounds; however, he handled me and my situation so well. He was open, caring, and responsive to my needs. I fully appreciate him because he was ultimately the one who got me back on track and pushed me to excel when I returned to work. I am where I am today because of him.

Pearl of Wisdom #10: Don't wait until something's wrong to familiarize yourself with your benefits. Review as much as you can until it's second nature. Whether it's your vision, medical, dental, or whatever your particular need is, make sure you're well-equipped and prepared for any and everything. Pay close attention to the long and short-term disability leave policy and what to do if you experience an illness. Please understand that sick leave benefits are not federally mandated or guaranteed. In addition, you may get paid while you're on leave; however, your job is not protected. By contrast, FMLA is a law that does protect your job during your absence. You must formally make the request in writing, submitting the proper paperwork to your employer.

WHEATGRASS JUICE

What a blessing that my sister is a healer who uses God's natural fruits and berries to combat illness. After hearing my diagnosis, she was very supportive, standing by my side when I needed her most. She never expressed that I shouldn't have surgery, but she vehemently rallied against chemotherapy. Before I knew any better, I was in agreement with her.

Prior to immersing myself in extensive research, my sister had me thinking I could change my diet, drink wheatgrass, and skip chemotherapy. In the 90s, my sister did two things that made me believe the natural approach could be a viable solution for me: She birthed my nephew naturally in a bathtub with a doula by her side. Secondly, she cured herself of a disease, by consuming the food of the Earth. Nothing synthetic, just herbs, supplements, vegan capsules, and vegetables.

Early on in my journey, there was a short period of time when I believed I didn't need chemotherapy.

After a few searches on cancer and chemotherapy, the strangest content started coming through my social media feeds. One post turned out to be a week-long, paid infomercial. I quickly gave my money to tune into this series, which detailed reasons *not* to subject the body to chemotherapy. I could eat fruits and berries, travel to Mexico to drink special combinations of teas and smoothies, consume apricot seeds, eat more fruits and berries, and many other things to be *CURED* of cancer.

Please know that I do believe in radical and spontaneous remission due to drastic diet changes. Back then, I just didn't see it as sustainable for me. The mind is a very powerful muscle; if I couldn't see and believe it happening for me, how could it be? There's one thing about life that I am sure of–what the mind can conceive, the body can and will achieve! My mind refused to believe what I'd heard, although I didn't completely discount it.

I need to point out the below information that comes up in most general research about fruits and vegetables. It's a part of healthy eating guidelines. **(Source: https://www.myplate.gov/)** On the negative side, you may hear there is too much natural sugar in fruits and that they must be carefully and thoroughly cleaned to avoid ingesting pesticides. However, on the flip side, fruits provide nutrients to maintain your health and body and may lower your risk for certain diseases. Clearly, one side looks better to deal with than the other.

From watching the infomercial, I took away many facts that I could use, like the benefits of plant based-lifestyles, avoiding hydrogenated fats, and concentrating on high-source nutrients. I also incorporated more exercise, yoga, and meditation into my routine. Truth be told, I already felt I was healthy doing all these things. But I still got cancer, so how could doing more make it go away?

I started second-guessing so many things. I hit the gym three times a week, and my eating habits could stand to be overhauled; however, I never missed scheduling or going to my doctor's appointments. This is primarily the reason I had so many second opinions regarding undergoing chemo and why I ultimately decided to go to a holistic facility. Following the first surgery that removed the cancer from my body, we knew it hadn't spread. I didn't believe I needed chemo, but I did. In the end, I incorporated a lot of what I'd seen in that infomercial. While I wanted to live, I knew I may falter. Taking wheatgrass every day wasn't it; the stuff is nasty! Some people tolerate it like candy in the flavor of Earth, but not me. Not to mention that halfway through my journey, according to the research my sister was doing, wheatgrass was now dangerous and shouldn't be ingested. I literally cannot make this stuff up.

Radical remission is a thing, but I knew I wasn't radical enough. It's important to know yourself. I'm a proponent of holistic methods, but please talk to your doctors. I had a team, and you need a team, too. Everyone was patient with me as I went through a period of indecision, but it's important to stick with your decisions once you make them and not be swayed. My sister was completely against chemo, yet she accompanied me to almost every one of my sessions without trying to dissuade me. If you have detractors in your life, you must figure out your *WHY*, your *YES*, and your *DESIRES* before inviting others in. Your journey is yours alone–they are just there for the ride. Remember, you are the captain, pilot, and CEO! Ultimately, I know I made the right decision for myself.

CHOOSING A CANCER TREATMENT CENTER

～～

My gynecologist is the reason I stand healthy today. Even after having a clean mammogram, she pressed me to get the sonogram and, ultimately, the biopsy that led to my diagnosis. She demanded I run, not walk, to get the medical attention I needed. Post diagnosis, it was she who directed me to which doctor was the best for me to connect with at the Bronx Center.

The young doctor recommended to me at the Bronx Center was pregnant. She was very nice, drew sketches of my breast, the milk ducts, the size and location of the cancer, and printed out a special study with facts and statistics for me to read. My journey was still in its infancy; the doctor seemed knowledgeable, but some of the information she relayed wasn't resonating in my spirit. I'm not sure how I was supposed to feel; however, I was unsettled. The plan she proposed to me didn't seem solid, so I contemplated my options. "You live in a city with a hospital that actually has a world-renowned name and care," I reminded myself. So, off to the large, fancy Manhattan Center I went.

Rashida took me to the Manhattan Center. Although it was a nicer facility, the welcoming committee left a lot to be desired. Donna called it the *Cadillac*, versus CTCA, which was the gold standard, or the *Rolls Royce*. The Manhattan Center was glaringly different from the Bronx Center. At first, it was the graham crackers in the waiting room for me. The sitting areas were different, inviting, comfortable, quiet, and uncrowded.

Nurses, doctors, and people in general seemed to be so much kinder at this center. I met with a surgeon who was a nice, knowledgeable man from Italy. Before I arrived at the Manhattan Center, I researched him and found out that he'd written extensive research papers on breast cancer and performed surgery for one of my best friend's mothers, which made me comfortable. I knew I was in the right place! Most of my diagnostic information was sent ahead of time to the doctor, and I brought additional notes and scans in case reinforcements were needed. Not only did he refer to the documents I brought with me, he included Rashida when advising what steps we were about to take.

The doctor made sure to mention that he was getting booked up and about to take vacation as the holidays were approaching. We all know how fear provokes us to make rash decisions, and it was no different for me. I immediately booked the surgery for Tuesday, November 29, 2016, with the reminder that even though I was having major breast cancer surgery, it was technically another appointment that could be canceled.

After scheduling the appointment, my doctor sent me for an MRI. He had everything from the Bronx Center; however, there were other factors he wanted to review prior to the surgery. I hated every minute of the exam! And why didn't I know until being contained in the MRI machine that I am claustrophobic? While I hated being confined in that small space, I knew it was needed for my care.

With the surgery now scheduled, I was locked in on the fancy Manhattan Center. Even though I didn't particularly like having to hustle to the city and hunt for parking, it was more important to me to be at what I then considered to be the upper echelon of cancer care hospitals in New York, so I was all in.

When I got back home and brought my caregivers up to speed, some of them were shocked that the surgery had been scheduled. Yes, this was happening, I was going with the flow, and everyone else needed to catch up. What I'd gone through over the last month made me keenly aware of myself and my surroundings, but after scheduling the surgery, something else clicked inside of me. I had to move with purpose and work to get my affairs in order.

My doctor gave me everything I needed to review and how to prepare leading up to the surgery, including filling out a living will and making sure my FMLA status at work was squared away. He also put in orders for me to have a radioactive solution injected into my body, to help him detect and remove some of my sentinel lymph nodes during the surgery.

I read the paperwork nonstop, a hundred times or more, to make sure I didn't miss a thing. The last thing I wanted was to jeopardize my health or do anything that would cause a problem on the day of my surgery. Back at work, I began the FMLA process. As much as I already knew, much of the cumbersome paperwork felt foreign to me, but I managed to fill it out and turn it in.

After the FMLA vendor got back to me, I had to have the documents signed by my doctor. All the back and forth took a week or so, but everything was getting done. By this time, I was running to more doctors, and bringing more people at work up to speed with what I was dealing with, which was important to solidify my time off. My coworkers were stepping up and much more supportive than I initially anticipated. As a mentor and facilitator in my group, I was documenting my steps to position everyone to proceed without me. Doing so in and of itself was a scary thought. I was preparing to be out for a few weeks, but what if something happened and I never came back? I tried not to allow my mind to venture to that thought too much, but it was undeniably present.

I also put measures into place for my family to make decisions on my behalf. I've always had a *will* in place, but I needed to implement the *living will* and *power of attorney*, to identify who would care for and speak for me in case I was alive, but incapacitated. With my being single and childless, I didn't want my mother to have to make these decisions. I designated my brother as the primary decision-maker and my sisters as secondary. It literally didn't matter who was listed in what place, though. My family would argue over a game of UNO, so I wouldn't expect anything less from them when it came to more important matters. I signed the paper-work, returned it to the hospital, and moved on.

Before the final task of going in for the sentinel node review the day before the surgery, I summoned my friends and family back together again to go to church and break bread. On November 27, 2016, my loved ones gathered at my church–First Baptist Church of East Elmhurst. There, they prayed with and for me and showered me with love. It was a special moment for me to have love poured into me, and a marvelous blessing. I was delighted that my pastor, Reverend Young, and the usher board were able to meet a lot of my family and friends. After service, we then walked up the block to my childhood home and broke bread together. It was a celebration of life in my honor, and my heart was overjoyed.

The next day, Rashida accompanied me to the city to have the radioactive seed implanted. Like my breast biopsy a month prior, this procedure was uncomfortable and outright painful! The sentinel node biopsy surgical procedure is used to determine whether cancer has spread beyond a primary tumor into the lymphatic system. I needed to have the procedure done before the first surgery so that once my body was opened, the doctor could decide how and what to operate on besides the breast. The actual node biopsy happened the next day during surgery; however, in order to prepare for it, I needed to have radioactive dye inserted prior. After having it done, I was required to carry a card noting I was radioactive. Even going to the airport for travel, I had to use caution–the fluid could set off alarms. I couldn't even hold babies or pets on my chest longer than 30-minute increments with the radioactive chemical in my body.

November 29, 2016. The morning after the smaller procedure to inject the radioactive fluids. My mother, brother, and I got up before dawn and headed out for the big surgery on the cold, dreary morning. It was so early when we left the house; the sky was still dark. By the time we got home, it was dark again. I don't recall being sad or scared; I just wanted the cancer out and to move on from it! Maybe it was naive of me to think one surgery and done. After all, I was armed with all those drawings from my doctors explaining the entire process. So many details hadn't registered, though. Perhaps I was being dense and illogical.

My brother is a police officer who drives fast and furiously. That morning, there was no speeding. No loud music distracting us. Nothing to make our mother say she was going to throw up. We weren't chipper or somber; we just were silent. Obviously, we were tired, but it was the mixed bag of emotions that had taken over.

We finally made it to the Manhattan Center, with no incidents, detours, or delays. The Manhattan Center had a solid, secure system. I signed in where we had to wait before signing in a second time on another floor. I was given an electronic name badge to wear, so I could easily be located anywhere in the hospital. My family could also check the board where my name was listed and showed how long I'd been in surgery. Right before they wheeled me back to the operating room, I took a selfie. All smiles, let's get 'er done.

After the procedure was complete, I woke up in the recovery room. The nurse asked me if I wanted to alert my family, but I asked her to hold off. I just needed some time to be alone and process what had just happened to me. The nurse granted me as much time as I needed. Alone in that room felt like a lifetime as I came to grips (yet again) with what I'd just endured. I was strong, but this was so much for one person! My attitude fluctuated between sadness, anger, frustration, and rage. Why was this happening to me! This horrible beast that tried to take my life had lost…it was a joy to have it snatched out! Finally, I pulled myself together and plastered my smile back on, even though it was fragile. That smile remained as I left the center.

Back at home, my boyfriend dropped by, along with friends. My nephews streamed in from work. I was sore and tired, but things were okay. My mother was waiting on me hand and foot, doing her best not to get on my nerves. It was an interesting two weeks of recovery: abdominal pain, a breast rash, swelling, and multiple calls to the doctors and nurses to see if any of it was normal.

I survived the two weeks and was anxious to follow up and get the results. Mom went with me to the appointment. *Did you get all of it?* was the first thought racing through my mind as we sat waiting. Then I wondered, *Can I go on vacation?* Boy, did I have my priorities out of order!

My doctor didn't hold any punches. A possible mastectomy, chemotherapy, and radiation. As he rattled off post-surgery treatment options, my soul was rattled. I thanked him for not glossing over the facts; I needed to know what I was facing in order to live. I probably should have taken a step back at that point. See, the surgery I had is known as a lumpectomy, on my right breast. A lumpectomy is considered a breast-conserving procedure. A *mastectomy* is the removal of the entire breast, nipple, areola, and all breast tissue, leaving the chest wall and muscle. The results of my genetic testing showed that I did not have a genetic disposition to cancer. Upon hearing this, I recalled reading the study that my doctor at the Bronx Center had given me, explaining the differences between a lumpectomy and mastectomy and how survival rates for my situation were relatively the same. Considering how early we discovered I had cancer, I elected to have the lumpectomy.

My mind was swirling. *So why are you telling me I need a mastectomy now?* I wondered.

My doctor said that my margins were not clear, that another surgery was needed, and based on how much needed to be removed, this time that a total right-side breast mastectomy and chemotherapy were necessary for my treatment.

Cancer centers assign a team of doctors for patients to see, so after sitting with the breast surgeon, I was referred to and met the medical oncologist, who explained the various chemotherapy drugs I could take. One of the medicines targeted seniors age 65 and older, which was less harsh. There were two other medications suggested to me as well: one contained a drug commonly known as the *red devil*–Adriamycin, which was extremely harsh. This medicine came highly recommended, but I refused to take it for two reasons. First, the infomercial flagged it as the worst medicine to take. Second, chemotherapy is toxic and can affect the heart. That sealed it for me. In 2009, my mother was diagnosed with a hereditary heart condition. I couldn't justify taking a drug that was supposed to help me beat cancer while destroying my heart.

You have cancer, Tricia. I understood that. Hell, I was living it. But I was unable to comprehend the pathology of it all. I had the best doctors at my disposal, yet somewhere along the line, someone forgot to tell me the experts needed to gauge the path forward based on what was seen during surgery. In my case, the pathology showed that even though the cancer was taken out, my margins were unclear, meaning the cancer was removed; however, it was present to the very edge. The point was to go back in and clean it all out. My doctor also said my best bet was to start chemo first, then go back in and completely clear it out...by removing my right breast. The good news was 11 nodes were removed from my underarm. They were clear, and the cancer had not spread. Still, there was the risk of developing lymphedema (swelling) from removing the nodes. There's probably a study regarding who's statistically prone to lymphedema and the varying amount of lymph nodes each of us has, but I'm not privy to it. Back then, I was so focused on the vacation I was excited to take, when it may have been in my best interest to focus on healing.

Due to the infomercial's emphasis on the harmful effects of chemotherapy, I was anti-chemo. Eventually,

I went on the hunt for more answers to help me decide my next steps. I was advised to get a second opinion, so I went back to the center that originally diagnosed me, but I didn't consult the breast surgeon whom I declined to perform my surgery. After speaking with a friend who was a doctor, I chose to meet with another oncologist. At the conclusion of that meeting, it was unanimous. Five different doctors who specialized in detecting and treating cancer said that because of the aggressive nature of the triple-negative breast cancer (TNBC), I'd been diagnosed with, chemotherapy was crucial.

Here's a bit of information regarding the type of breast cancer I was diagnosed with. There are three receptors that breast cancer can have: positive/negative estrogen hormone, negative/positive progesterone hormone, and a positive/negative protein called HER2. You can have all positive receptors, a variation of positive negative, or all negative. For breast cancer with a positive receptor, there are hormone therapies that can kill the cancer without chemotherapy; however, for patients with triple-negative breast cancer, options are limited. In 2016, chemotherapy and radiation were still the gold standard of care.

Even though I wasn't in agreement with this plan, I knew all the physicians wouldn't steer me wrong. This was it; chemo was about to be my new reality. But once the treatments began, who was going to care for me? *The whole person?* I emphasize the whole person because of the toxic nature of chemotherapy. Yes, the treatment kills the cancerous cells that do not follow healthy cell patterns, rapidly dividing and doing their own thing. But, chemotherapy treatments also kill off good cells in the body, which made me explore a mixture of Western and Eastern medicine to alleviate this.

There was so much to digest with chemotherapy, which I hadn't dealt with before. For one thing, because of chemo, I now had to consider saving my eggs. Coupled with my age and previous issues with my lady parts, once I began treatment, my fertility was going to be affected. Although I felt like my eggs were already scrambled with cheese, my mate at the time thought we should look into preserving my eggs.

Additionally, the mention of having a mastectomy was stuck in the back of my mind. The doctors wanted me to get started on chemotherapy right away, so conserving my breast and eggs was an afterthought. As a project manager, I appreciate having all the scenarios and answers up front, so I can put a viable plan into place; however, I was starting to learn that you cannot *project manage* breast cancer. I had to take a step back and listen to the advice of the doctors before making any moves.

MY FRIED EGGS

I was halfway over 40 when I was diagnosed, wasn't thinking about children, and clinging to a fragile, mediocre relationship. Was going through the egg-preserving process on top of everything else even worth it? Years ago, a married friend told me never bring a child into a broken relationship thinking it will make things better because it won't. Truthfully, that's why I'd never had a child all these years–most of my relationships were nothing more than space fillers. Years of therapy have taught me that I was never taught how to love and create a lasting relationship. Yet there I was, making decisions about the rest of my life, and this part of my future focused squarely on love and relationships.

I'm going to be real. Preparing to fight for my life shoved saving my eggs to the bottom of my list of priorities. However, a lot of things happened that made me take it into serious consideration. A friend brought it up to me, my doctor explained what would happen to my reproductive system, the genetics team asked me about having children, a nurse navigator recommended I at least look into it, and my mate said, "Why not try?" Each of these factors played a tremendous part in entertaining it as a viable option for my future. Let's have a moment of truth here: The only reason I truly agreed to move forward with harvesting my eggs was because I found out that as a cancer patient, the cost of the process was severely discounted.

The day of the harvesting, my mate went with me. The medical staff asked questions, I answered, they drew blood, and the procedure began. I honestly don't know how much I wanted to do this because it's the part of my journey that I remember the least about. I've blocked most of it out; it was excruciatingly painful, both mentally and physically. I went through the motions and showed up to have my uterus surveyed at the crack of dawn, all for nothing.

No viable eggs were produced.

The most I can remember is paying the nurse who lived in Dobbs Ferry to go to her house, where she administered shots in my stomach or thigh. Once I grew tired of driving all the way out there, I consulted with one of my sorority sisters–a nurse who lived much closer to me. She agreed to administer the shots, which worked well for a while, until I grew tired of that too.

Finally, I realized that no one could take my pain away or go through the process for me, so I elected to administer the shots myself. In retrospect, perhaps my partner and I could have navigated the process together in love. If we had, maybe something real would have been conceived from it. Unfortunately, we were not mentally prepared for that. This process should have brought us closer together, allowed us to dive deeper into our relationship, and work out our problems. Yet, we floated through it with zero connection to each other.

Our relationship lacked color. Zeal. Excitement. All of the dating shows I frequently watch usually showcase a couple doing daring and exciting things to help them bond; I'd say the reverse is also true. The valley can be scary, but going through it together helps couples bond. We just couldn't get there.

It's important to note that I don't blame my mate. I played a huge part in our demise by misrepresenting myself and my true feelings the entire time we were together. Early on in our relationship (probably too early), I asked him about kids. He didn't seem to be serious about wanting any, and I wasn't pressed to have children, either. It was fine at first; however, it was years before turning 40 and being diagnosed with cancer. Eventually, I came to see that what I wanted didn't match what he wanted.

Given what he'd told me before, I was shocked that he wanted me to try to conserve my eggs. The sentiment was empty, though. And it was frankly too little, too late. My mind and my heart weren't fully invested in the process. I was stuck on years of disagreements and letdowns. Again, not placing full blame because I played a large supporting role in this. Our relationship suffered because I hadn't learned how to truly forgive and live in the present.

There were a few times my mate refused to come with me to an appointment because we had an argument the night before. I got fed up. Told him that the months ahead of me were going to be difficult, and if he couldn't handle it, he just needed to go away! I needed a strong team, and he wasn't a star player. And just like that…he stopped showing up at home for days at a time. A mutual friend of ours had to talk him into coming back. The scenario wasn't anything new to our relationship; I always clamored for him, or others had to pressure him, but he never returned to me on his own accord. It was always under duress. There were so many things that I was hell-bent on being upset about, that I forgot to extend both of us grace.

In the end, the process did not work. I don't know what it was, but there are a couple of things that come to mind. I wasn't completely engaged, my body was taxed, I was stressed, and I didn't want to bring a child into this crazy world in the first place. I was more anxious about moving forward in my cancer journey. The two months I spent trying to save my eggs was just a pitfall along the way. I may never truly know what could have been or why it all went south, but I do know that I gave it my best at the time. In the end, I have to believe that God made this decision for me, and I have no regrets. It just wasn't for me.

In recently speaking with other survivors, some of the women mentioned *Lupron* to me. I was upset because a few short years ago, I'd never heard of it. It's a drug that can be taken monthly and helps maintain the menstrual cycle following chemotherapy. According to Drugs.com, Lupron shuts off the body's normal egg development, controls hormones, and helps improve the number and quality of eggs available for fertilization. Again, everything around this time is a blur; I'm not sure what I was taking, but I would've remembered Lupron.

After a time, I got real quiet with myself. For years I'd been okay with it all, yet there I was, wondering, *Why not me?* When I think about how on most days, I don't have time to move from my desk, eat a decent meal, exercise or get enough sleep, I quickly snap out of it. I thoroughly enjoy my life as it is–if a child was a part of my world, I'd figure it all out, but the cards I was dealt led me down a different path. I choose to be happy where I am. Breakfast is my favorite meal of the day, and I will continue having my eggs scrambled with cheese, please.

Pearl of Wisdom #11: Ladies, I implore you to freeze your eggs prior to experiencing reproductive challenges. The brunt of the cost is in saving the eggs for countless years; however, harvesting them provides viable alternatives if you have issues conceiving. More African-American women are delaying having children until they find the right man or get where they want in their careers. So, saving your eggs at a young age only makes sense.

CHOOSING A CANCER TREATMENT CENTER - PART 2

~~~

As part of coming to terms with taking chemotherapy, I gathered opinions from a few doctors and friends. I didn't really have any friends who'd been through this journey, or at least none who had spoken to me personally about it. The immense pressure of not having a true confidante made me feel so alone. The first surgery was done; I'd gone on a luxury vacation and taken the time to save my eggs, even though it failed. Now it was time to begin chemotherapy and get everything else back on track.

I entered 2017 with plans upon plans. Enduring six months of chemotherapy and radiation was going to take a toll on my body and mental health. For that reason, I wanted to get started and past it as soon as possible.

One day, a sorority sister put me in touch with a survivor friend of hers, who was God sent! A two-time breast cancer survivor, she consistently texted and called me, pouring valuable information I needed to know in me. She took the time to explain her journey and how she survived to me, putting my anxiety somewhat at ease. Much like me, she desired a holistic approach to conquering cancer. On her accord, she explained that she'd been flown to Illinois and was seen at a center that took care of the whole body.

So far, at both centers where I'd been treated, no one discussed Eastern medical philosophies. The options presented to me were unfulfilling. What I was missing was a doctor who treated the *whole* person. I was already into holistic medicine, so when she explained other supplements and innovative treatments she'd used (such as Vitamin C infusions and Mistletoe Therapy), I was hooked! It was all so intriguing; after all the negative press/information I'd consumed regarding chemotherapy, here was someone who'd successfully undergone it.

The naturopathic doctor I'd been seeing for years resided in Connecticut. One year when treating my finger, which had become infected at the nail salon, she gave me a tincture with instructions to drop a few drops on my finger daily. My doctor literally cured my nail infection without antibiotics. I was in shock, but that was her craft. While in her care over the years, I've also completed three thermograms: heat-sensitive photographs taken with sophisticated infrared cameras. Potential problem areas are indicated by abnormal temperature readings. **(Source: https://integratedhealthcenteron-line.com/breast-health/)**

My thermogram showed a 3 in my right breast and a 1-2 in my left breast. A 3 means preventative actions should be taken to prevent the issue from turning into something bigger. I opted to face it head-on, taking supplements and improving my diet, although I was inconsistent with eating better. I didn't fully understand the power of the information I was armed with then, but I do now. Obviously, we are here today because I still got breast cancer; however, I think I was better positioned to fight it due to my diligence and knowledge I obtained years prior. I was and still remain a worrier, meticulously investigating everything I notice going on in my body—as I should. I don't race to the doctor for every little thing, but I do monitor any abnormalities for a week or two. It's important to watch without stressing, which can cause another set of issues.

As you can see, I've been trying to cure myself of various things for many years. I was very skeptical about flying out of town for treatments, and was overwhelmed with information. However, everything my soror's friend told me was right up my alley. I was all in, though I wondered how I would accomplish this feat. That's when she gave me the magical advice: "You don't need to fly to Illinois, Tricia. There's a center in Philadelphia." That did it for me. Without delay, I called CTCA to find out what they offered. A pleasant man answered my call; I believe he was a survivor. He spoke to me for about 30 minutes before advising he or someone else would call back. Thankfully, they did.

CTCA didn't accept my insurance, which scared me. Treating cancer is extremely expensive, but I knew what I wanted. In the end, my insurance situation was worked out. I was excited because the center had everything I needed under one roof and treated the whole person. What distinguishes a place? I'm here to tell you that most cancer centers have the same basic standard of care. Keep in mind that while the disease itself is fast-changing, treating cancer also has a standard of care. The facility you choose and its staff is where the rubber meets the road.

CTCA was like the bar on *Cheers*–everyone knew your name and was always glad you came! Sometimes, I thought the entire staff took a swig of helium daily to keep them so happy. It didn't matter why; I was bursting with gratitude for the pure joy my family, friends, and I experienced each time we entered CTCA's doors. They greet you, take your coat and bags, and if you arrive via any mass transportation, you're usually picked up from the terminal in a limousine. (Later on, as costs were cut, it became nice sedans and SUVs). One thing that stood out for me was how super friendly the drivers were, how they opened doors and greeted you by name.

Even if they didn't know your name, the staff always smiled and recognized our faces. Everyone was engaged, warm, and inviting, and the spacious waiting rooms were accommodating. The recliners were comfortable; since there was so much to do, the wait never felt as long as it really was. Whether it be jigsaw puzzles, drawings to color or paint by number, a librarian passing out books to the patients, or popular shows playing on the TVs, our minds were occupied. And don't forget the snacks–there was plenty of ginger ale, water, graham crackers, or saltines readily available when we wanted it. Speaking of food, the cafeteria was well-stocked, and the food was provided at a low cost.

I've never seen *Alice in Wonderland,* but CTCA made it feel like I was there. I never wanted for anything! There was a small activity center, a spa, hair salon, and the grounds outside were beautiful. Aside from my doctors, I was able to see a masseuse, hairdresser, pharmacist, acupuncturist, nutritionist, naturopathic practitioner, chiropractor, yoga or music therapy instructor, support groups, a pastor, and go to church, all on-site.

Out of four different cancer centers that I've been to, hands down, CTCA is one of the best places on Earth for whole-body health. I wouldn't change my time at CTCA for anything; I highly recommend anyone in need of cancer care to check them out. Although the Philadelphia, Pennsylvania location was later shut down, there are three other locations in the contiguous United States.

It wasn't until the very end, when CTCA was closing, and a number of services were cut, that I had complaints. I imagine the other locations are still thriving; however, Philly was my location of choice. I thank them for the life-saving techniques and services that they provided, not just for me, but the countless others they served.

THE ROLLS ROYCE OF CANCER TREATMENT CENTERS

My first visit to CTCA was on February 2, 2017. My mate was going to take me, but my brother said family should be there. Admittedly, I shouldn't have excluded my mate, but I was too weak and feeble-minded to understand what counting him out would do to our relationship. Nonetheless, it was my brother Kerry and I who took the road trip to Philly. When we arrived, I underwent a two-day evaluation to determine whether or not I'd be accepted as a patient. I was nervous but ready for the 100th opinion I'd received. Mentally, I already knew what needed to be done; however, I wanted to hear the CTCA staff's perspective.

I was greeted by the director of patient relations, who took me on a brief tour of the center's ground level before handing me a thin binder to keep my notes and business cards I received from the doctors. He ushered me past the large, stunning fish tanks as we ventured onto the 5th floor. Immediately, I was shown to the patient evaluation room, where I sat half the day, medical personnel streaming in and out of the room to see me. Having them come to me instead of bouncing around the center was one of the best parts of the long wait. It didn't hurt that I was also served a modest meal of my choice.

My brother, on the other hand, was knocked out. I was disappointed but not angry. After all, I was my brother's second job. Every couple of weeks, he and my other caregivers got off work on a Wednesday or Thursday, then we hit the road straight to CTCA. After the first time we went, the visits cost more energy and emotional work than any of us anticipated. Having reinforcements who had my back was a tremendous help; I may have been sick, but I was never alone. No matter the day or the appointment, passing the time laughing and talking with others always helped.

I'm struggling to recall how a college friend and sorority sister ended up going to my initial visit, but she was right there, supporting me. Considering we hadn't spoken in over a year, it was odd; however, this particular friend and I always fell right back on track in our friendship, no matter how much time had passed. We reminisced, joked, laughed about the past, and caught up with how things were going since she had moved south, before circling back to the visit to CTCA.

She sat in on a doctor's visit with Kerry; if I recall correctly, the appointment was for genetics counseling. Kerry and I are seven years apart and never attended any of the same schools, but at the same time, he's familiar with many of my friends, and I know many of his. Those two sat in that room cutting up! I was almost mad, but how could I be? The appointments were tough, but I was supported the entire way. They needed a break from the heaviness, just as I did.

We all had lunch together before my friend left. She and I never spoke much about my journey after that day, but I was excited to see her. Without a doubt, I knew then, and I know now that she has my back, and I have hers forever and a day without hesitation.

My second day at the center was the tougher of the two since the first day was mostly filled with PAs asking what seemed to be random questions. Now I know nothing is random during this journey; however, having my pathology report, scans from my mammogram, biopsy, MRI, and my surgery back in November 2016 sent ahead of my arrival helped immensely. But there was still a lot more to do.

Over the course of two days, I met with the medical oncologist, breast surgeon, radiation oncologist, and geneticist. I walked the halls, met other staff members, learned more about CTCA, and immersed myself in the culture. CTCA was such a caring place; I loved having access to everything I needed under one roof. They didn't limit what they told me to only what I wanted to hear, but what I *needed to know*, in a sensitive, empowering manner.

While I knew chemotherapy was inevitable, I was determined to avoid dealing with the harshest drugs. When I was diagnosed, the cancer was only at Stage 1 - .08 millimeters in diameter, which was a good thing. Might I add the cancer was literally removed, but I did not want the *red devil* chemotherapy that could affect my heart when I may have already been compromised by Mom's hereditary heart issue. Later, I learned that my mother's condition was not passed down to me; however, it's still something I had to be cognizant of following chemotherapy, which can have long-term effects, like COVID.

Many statistics I've studied state that taking this drug gives patients a 5% probability of contracting leukemia. Having to consider one bad issue over the next is daunting. Prescriptions typically detail the benefits of taking the prescribed medication while noting the risks as well. I was extremely pleased that my new medical team agreed with me on a few things: I didn't need the *red devil*, and it appeared I wouldn't need a total mastectomy of the right breast! Yes, chemotherapy was still on the plate as well as a second surgery, but nothing as extreme as we initially thought.

At this point, it was four months since I'd been diagnosed. Genetic testing was complete, I had tried conserving my eggs, and I was cleared by a cardiologist to move forward with chemotherapy. With everything they presented and how comfortable they made me, I decided to continue my care with CTCA. Without satellite offices in New York, this meant traveling back and forth to the center for my appointments via car or Amtrak. I was overjoyed they accepted my case. This was the place I wanted to be; if it's possible to be happy to start cancer care, I was.

THE RED HEAD WITH THE BANJO

The first visit to CTCA had all of us ready to wet our pants. My brother, sister, and friend kicked off my chemotherapy journey with me. The thing is, we weren't by ourselves–we were in a waiting area with another family, and none of us were able to contain our hysteria. Every so often, we'd see a doctor with red hair who carried all types of things, including a banjo. Had she not been wearing a white coat, freely walking in and out of offices, and smiling like she owned the world, I might've mistaken her for a homeless person.

Obviously, the doctor sensed us gawking at her, so she approached us between appointments, asking if we'd like to observe what she did. Of course, we did! We followed her, laughing under our breath, bumping each other as we walked, clueless as to what we were walking into. The doctor's name was Allie–Mind, Body, Medicine/Music Therapist.

Dr. Allie carefully explained her job to us, but we still didn't get it. The explanation was elusive at best. I soon learned that while Dr. Allie's methods were interactive and innovative, the sessions were more about how she made you feel or how you made yourself feel with her guidance.

To me, Dr. Allie helped patients get their minds right. She taught me how to center myself with deep breathing, how to stretch and correctly perform yoga positions, calm my nerves by looking within and using a sound drum, which was pivotal. My sun sign is Pisces; I'm most comfortable and relaxed when I am in or near bodies of water, which typically happens when I'm on vacation. For me, water equates to relaxation and joy. The sound drum took me to that place.

Meditation was also a part of Dr. Allie's practice. I'm not sure I ever got any of this correct, but I kept going back because I always left Dr. Allie's sessions feeling better. I really adored my time with her, and still perform bits and pieces of what she taught me today. Had I continued the doctor's practices, I think my health would be a million times better. Dr. Allie was one of the reasons CTCA sometimes felt like I was visiting an oasis. There, I was able to put my everyday life aside and focus on what was most important to me—my health. It's not always realistic to always do that, but as I write this book, I realize that I can carve out 10-15 minutes a day to implement the techniques I gained from Dr. Allie into my everyday routine.

While some of the things Dr. Allie did (and frankly, how she looked) were often laughable, she was far from the entertainment. For me, Dr. Allie was one of the prized possessions of CTCA. Every time I entered the building, I wanted Dr. Allie on my schedule. She provided a different outlook on what was happening to me and was the break I needed from the stream of doctors potentially delivering bad news.

Aside from learning yoga and meditation, Dr. Allie used a banjo for music therapy. Music has the ability to take us away, transforming us from what we're feeling to seeing a different perspective. Dr. Allie didn't play the banjo for me, but during the holidays, when the pianist was playing near the Christmas tree, she occasionally accompanied him. It was so beautiful; the patients gathered around the fireplace, minds totally adrift, lost in the music.

Dr. Allie played music from her phone during our sessions. Melodic, calming music as if we were relaxing in a spa or therapy. She recommended that I research meditation music, which I took her up on. I found similar music, but you know how a DJ mixes music for you to dance to all night? Well, my meditation music never quite came out like Dr. Allie's. I've since discovered the group *Beautiful Chorus*, whose music metaphorically transcends darkness to light for me.

Dr. Allie literally transformed every space she was in. The harsh lights were lowered, and the scent of glorious essential oils permeated the room, creating a peaceful atmosphere. Upon arrival, you may feel agitated, but once stepping inside, your spirit comes alive, and you leave feeling awakened. Dr. Allie's nurturing nature calmed my storm when I needed it most. Her tender care helped adult cancer patients relax, relate, and release on their own. Find yourself a Dr. Allie, or become her to strengthen yourself. All you need is a designated relaxation space–even if it's only inside your mind, as you slowly inhale and exhale.

Dr. Allie taught me to relax. During your cancer journey, you cannot run from your sickness or your feelings. It's important to sit with both and work through it all. Even on a regular day, growing up, I was nervous and anxious about everything. Dr. Allie's practices helped me more than I initially realized. Sometimes, I have trouble sleeping, so I use the grounding techniques of the moon salutation that Dr. Allie showed me. I don't move swiftly through the positions; however, I intentionally move slowly, feeling every position. Taking my time helps me check my form and prepare for rest.

Dr. Allie left CTCA after meeting the love of her life. (I believe she moved to Europe). She's one of the people that I miss the most from CTCA, but I'm grateful for what she taught and did for me, and the time we had together.

Pearl of Wisdom #12: During your cancer journey, take time to slow down and practice self-care. Journal, listen to music, meditate, diffuse soothing essential oils, or do what makes you happy. You can also visit my website for suggestions on how to engage in self-care. Remember, calming your mind and spirit is free medicine.

COLD CAP DECISION

~~~

A Black woman's hair is her crown. It's an integral part of her appearance, showing who she is and speaking before she does. Hair has been and will probably always be an important backdrop to my life. It's a character on its own.

Growing up, I'd always been self-conscious about my hair. From my pigtail days in grade school to being called Celie (from *The Color Purple*) while in college because of how I *styled* my hair, people have always defined me by my kinks and coils. Society has ingrained in us that long, straight European tresses are preferred to short, coily, and kinky. Some of us have no choice, but we went through the arduous task of trying to get what has been considered the standard.

For years, my hair was relaxed by the same stylist of over twenty years. Every two weeks, we had an appointment, or I'd visit weekly for special events. Talking and laughing with my salon family while my hair was being done was time well spent. When I was a kid, I couldn't participate in grown folks' conversations, but now that I was an adult, it was on!

I spent countless hours at that salon, getting my hair and nails done. For the most part, I didn't get super elaborate styles, just a wash and set with 30 minutes of conditioning time. Sitting under the dryer was the worst! It felt like my brain cells were burning. Once I ditched those methods, I started getting braids–a style I loved but hated the process, especially the pain of the stylist pulling my hair too tight. Today, braids are back in style; however, now I have a voice, and I'm able to stop the braider from pulling the braids so darn tight to my scalp.

Then there were the weaves. Honey, when I finally got some real money flowing in, you couldn't tell me I wasn't Mary J. Blige with my straight, blonde weaves installed with the best human hair mixture. My stylist was from London and was obsessed with using the best of everything. She only used Black-owned hair care products, like Dudleys. I believe my stylist knew the Dudley family personally and refused to let me buy weaving hair from the regular beauty supply stores. No ma'am, she sent me to Bobbie's Hair World. The amount of money I was spending on my hair and the hours spent in the salon were atrocious...we were doing things for the 'gram before Instagram was a thing.

Thinking of the massive hours I spent holed up in a salon and the hundreds I spent on my hair, it was easy for me to say, *"Man, if I get cancer, I would chop it all the way off!"* Yes, there was a time before cancer when I said IF I ever were to get cancer, I would have no problem cutting my hair off as it would save me time and money. Who knew that would become a reality?

While hair was very important to me, and I took care of it as best I could, my hair wasn't in the best state. At times my crown went through horrible phases; I experienced hair loss due to trauma and emotional and physiological stress. Years before cancer, I was experiencing serious hair shedding. I remember staying overnight at the home of an ex, only to wake up the next morning with hair everywhere! I warned him that my hair had shed and the floor needed to be swept; he behaved as if I'd done this on purpose. That's when I knew I wasn't the only one and never went back there.

Another time, I walked into the salon, dejected. I was wearing my favorite old gray sweats, a random t-shirt, and sneakers. Not a cute look at all. My stylist didn't say a word until I plopped in her chair. She lit into me! "You might come here to get glamorous, but happiness and beauty is still an inside job," she fussed. She didn't care a thing about my man problems, either. "I don't care what's going on with him; you cannot be defeated. Even if you're down, you don't live in that state long, and definitely don't come outside looking like that!"

That was just one of the talks my stylist and I had over the years. She consistently spoke to my spirit, like many of the people on my team. It was like walking into a therapy session; I always knew my people by the quality of the time we spent together. My years at the salon were some of the best learning opportunities.

Throughout the years, the ups and downs continued with my tresses and my relationships. In 2011, I attempted the big chop. It was bad. I had broken up with a boyfriend and wanted to start fresh. My stylist asked if I was crazy and refused to cut it. I swear, we almost had a *Waiting to Exhale* moment right then and there. If she didn't cut it, I was going to! Reluctantly (and somewhat grudgingly), my stylist eventually cut my hair, although she left more hair than I wanted on my head before she colored it. I loved it, but we lightened it too much. Peering at the pictures of that fresh look today, all I see is how brave and bold I was to do it. But it didn't suit me.

I'm not sure who besides me sits around thinking about these things, but I always loved my hair and wanted more of it. Actually, I wanted hair like my mother's. I was always threatening to cut it all off, so it could finally grow in fresh after years of bad manipulation. That way, it had the chance to grow in like Mom's. That odd time in 2011 aside, I never quite pulled the trigger, though I maintained zero hesitation, repeating that if I ever got cancer, I was going to do it. Five years later, I was now apprehensive about losing my hair.

This was a concern for me because the doctor explained the treatments and how my body would be affected. My friend Adrienne honed in on two things that stood out: *fertility and hair*. Adrienne is five years younger than me, and we'd been friends for about three years before becoming sorority sisters. She's a bit of a fashionista and brilliant; I consider her my personal Google. Adrienne had been researching hair-saving techniques for such a time as this...she intentionally started researching this specifically for me. Just like that, I was sold. All the talk about chopping my hair off if I got cancer was out the window. With so many things about to change in my life (mainly, my appearance), I wanted something about me to stay the same.

So what was this thing that could help me save my hair? Not many people, in general, used it consistently, and there weren't enough African-American, natural, kinky-headed sisters out here doing it. Adrienne did most of the initial research before I took over. I reached out to a sister with a strong internet presence regarding Black hair care who had breast cancer. When we spoke, she told me she'd cut her hair and nursed it back to health. I searched high and low but couldn't find anyone who looked like me that used the cold caps.

Still determined, I found a cold cap distributor and contacted them, inquiring whether they accepted insurance or not. At this point, the big chop was looking like a more viable solution due to the astronomical cost I faced.

One day before the procedures began, I nearly had a nervous breakdown when I stepped out of the shower and glared at myself in my full-length mirror. So much was about to change in my world, and I didn't know how to handle it. I groped my breast, wishing things could stay the same. Ultimately, I decided to go for the cold caps. After submitting the initial payment of $400, I was obligated to pay $333 a month for the next four months. The process involved cooling the caps the night before with dry ice, which added an additional cost that my brother paid for. It was all so much! Trekking to treatments out of state, and now there were the cold caps and dry ice to deal with. I was getting more stressed by the minute.

My decisions didn't only affect me. It meant transporting myself and three other adults to Philadelphia, cooling the caps for at least 12 hours before using them, and getting them to Philadelphia, too. All this while keeping ourselves safe from the dry ice fumes, which can be damaging to the nervous system or burn if touched by bare hands.

This wasn't a smidge of dry ice, either. It was pounds! We drove to CTCA with the windows rolled down in the middle of winter. We were so nervous that we once slept with the ice cooler outside the hotel room. After that, we were afraid it would get stolen, so we ended up leaving the caps inside the cooler in the car. The caps had to be worn 30 minutes prior to my chemotherapy starting and throughout the duration of my IV drip, then for two more hours. In all, I froze my hair follicles and entire head for upwards of seven hours. I'd come full circle from burning my brain cells under a hair dryer for hours to freezing them.

The entire situation with the caps turned out to be more of a chore for my family, beyond transporting them. All eight of the caps were numbered; there was an entire process of using and rotating the caps in and out of the cooler to keep them cool enough for the maximum amount of time. Timing was everything–opening the cooler, checking the temperature with an infrared thermometer, removing the cap I was wearing, replacing the new cap's packing, and putting the old cap back in the cooler. It was all so tedious, yet each step was vital in maintaining the effectiveness of the process. My mother, brother Kerry, sister Loretta, and friend Donna were all part of this whole sting operation; I couldn't have done it without each of them.

Have I mentioned that the caps needed to be changed every 30 minutes? My friend and family literally left their full-time jobs to cater to me and this unpaid assignment, which was mentally and physically taxing. Donna and Loretta usually fit me with the caps, and Kerry used the special gloves to open the cooler, fish out a cap and bury the old one.

Late at night, when we'd settled back in the hotel, Donna switched the caps at least three more times. As I watched her, it never failed–I teared up. I was tired, cold and hated those caps! I was over the entire process and didn't want to do it anymore!

Back in Queens, my mother helped out with cooking, helping with other daunting tasks I couldn't get to, and served as basic moral support, which eased the stress for my siblings and me. We were such a big group with so many moving parts that the center gave me the coveted personal suite on occasion, although I was in the general population for the majority of my visits. I think the staff was trying to relieve my family and me of some of the stress. It was hard, but at least we still had our joy. We did the best we could to be strong while still enjoying life along the way. I believe that's why they intentionally placed me in general population at times—so others could be inspired by our process and interactions.

Now if you're keeping track, I opted to be treated at CTCA-Philadelphia and to use chemotherapy cold caps to preserve my hair. Okay, back to my family. I know they thought going out to Philly and putting all of us through the process with the cold caps was insane, but they never second-guessed my decisions to my face. Hell, my sister, Lorretta, was an integral part of the process! She told me she'd never subject herself to chemotherapy and didn't want me to either, but she stood by my side as one of my biggest cheerleaders. FYI, the cold caps did save my hair, but it works better on straight European hair.

Pearl of Wisdom #13: I want to note that many people talk about the hair on your head that is lost. So that you are not shocked, I want to alert you that other hair on your body, like your eyebrows, lashes, underarms, and pubic hair, are also lost during chemotherapy. Try to prepare yourself mentally and develop a beauty routine that helps you to still feel beautiful.

WRITE THE LETTERS

Let's talk about saving money. Battling cancer isn't a volunteer service for anyone involved, especially the patients themselves. It's expensive, sudden, and most people aren't prepared for it. There are ways to save money, but you have to put in the work. Start by reaching out to sponsors and donors. Write the letters, fill out the applications and call the decision-makers. My financial advisor constantly advises me to put away at least six months' worth of money in an emergency fund. I must admit that I was nowhere near that amount at the start of my journey. Due to some decisions I made along the way, I needed much more money, but thankfully, I had gainful employment with great insurance.

During my first visit to the Manhattan Center, I was passed a book of resources that included financial resources. For the longest time, I skipped over that part because the insurance I had was accepted in Manhattan. After making the switch to CTCA, I discovered my insurance wasn't accepted, and the chemotherapy cold caps weren't covered, either. This is where the other resources came into play.

The most time-consuming part of this portion of the journey was scouring the resources for what's being offered and how my situation fit in. Your facility should give you a similar list to what I have posted in the *Appendix*. Listen, no one is handing out $100 dollar bills on the street corner; however, the government and other various organizations have designated funds specifically for cancer patient care, but you must exercise due diligence in searching for it.

CTCA had its own program. Once I was approved, I was able to receive funding that I was able to apply yearly for. That worry aside, now I had to tackle ancillary details, like the fact that the chemo cold caps were considered a *want* as opposed to a need. That scared me. I desperately wanted to keep my hair–it was a part of me. But the cost to keep it was astronomical. There are two things I did that helped me along this part of my journey.

I conferred with a couple of close friends, who recommended I write letters to different agencies for help. Being vulnerable about your finances with others is scary; I don't like rejection, and it's hard to open up when you're afraid to fail and not get what you've asked for. But when you have a village like mine, you know your friends and family will be there to help you pick up the pieces and win.

Soon after sharing my dilemma with the agencies, I was given a card during a chapter meeting, which I still have to this day. It had a wad of cash in it and was signed by over 20 people to be put towards the cost of my chemo cold caps. My friends and family raised funds for me; I was speechless. Time and again throughout my journey, I was given money that I could never ever repay; keeping count of it all was impossible. Feeling indebted to others is a hard pill to swallow; however, I accepted my blessing and prayed that if I'm ever given the opportunity to do the same, I'd be able to without hesitation.

Without knowing the fundraiser was happening, I wrote an angry letter to my insurance company expressing my dissatisfaction that the cold caps weren't covered and demonstrating my need for help. After months of back and forth showing proof, receipts, and even pictures of myself using the caps, I was partially reimbursed.

Again, keeping copies of everything is paramount. That's what helped me win my case. Tracking my medical expenses and keeping receipts had a major impact on the outcome. Most organizations want to see that you specifically invested a certain amount of dollars into specific areas of concern. In short, you have to demonstrate the need. I'll also add that I'd seen a few doctors who didn't accept the insurance; however, I was able to show how I was directly impacted by cancer and had some costs subsidized.

Keep in mind that if you can prove a certain amount of your income is going toward medical expenses, it counts as a deduction on your taxes. Based on my decisions, my medical expenses increased, but my tax professional helped me recoup some of it. I wasn't happy with the amount that I was reimbursed, but I was thankful. Still, it felt like I was draining money faster than it came in.

For a short while, when I was on disability, my salary dropped to 60%. I thought I was going to break! Luckily, there was a mistake found on my paperwork that initiated the decrease, and I was reimbursed in back pay. It came weeks later; however, it came at a time when I was pinching pennies, so I was grateful.

My hope is that being transparent about my journey will give you some of the relief you need right now. There is support out there for you, and it's not always financial. I've come across legal support and services through various programs and organizations that are extremely helpful. (Please refer to the *Appendix*). When I've written letters in the past, expressing my displeasure with a product or how a worker in a store represented the store, I didn't always receive a response. I was persistent in taking the steps that would give me the satisfaction I wanted. Today, the process has been streamlined to make things easier. All you have to do is complete the application or write a short story detailing your needs. Keep in mind whoever's in charge only wants the facts, so just give it to them.

Pearl of Wisdom #14: Apply, apply, apply, appeal, appeal, appeal! Don't take "NO" for an answer; keep appealing! Many patients get frustrated and cut the process short. Those are the ones who end up paying out of pocket or being denied life-sustaining services. Your first appeal is with the insurance company. If you're denied again, it's time to appeal to a state agency or an independent medical review organization.

FIRST CHEMO TREATMENT

～～

As per *Mayo Clinic,* "Chemotherapy is a drug treatment that uses powerful chemicals to kill fast-growing cells in your body. Though chemotherapy is an effective way to treat many types of cancer, chemotherapy treatment also carries a risk of side effects. Some chemotherapy side effects are mild and treatable, while others can cause serious complications."

According to *Cancer.org,* "Chemotherapy drugs are considered to be hazardous to people who handle them or come into contact with them. For patients, this means the drugs are strong enough to damage or kill cancer cells. But this also means the drugs can be a concern for others who might be exposed to them."

This is why there are safety rules and recommendations for people who handle chemo drugs. Chemotherapy is a serious matter; I was terrified but knew that it was an important part of my treatment plan.

My first chemotherapy appointment was scheduled for February 17, 2017. The plan was for me to wrap up work at home, have everything packed, and my friend Donna would pick me up and take me to Mom's house in Queens, so I could hug and kiss her before hitting the road with Kerry, Loretta, and Donna. Our goal was to depart by 6:30 and arrive in Philly around 9 p.m.

None of which happened.

Well, the first trip was absolutely haywire! The way Donna tells it is absolutely hilarious. I was in my house finishing up work and hadn't packed a thing. Clothes were everywhere! As soon as Donna walked in the house, her eyes bucked. She knew that I don't keep a messy house and how generally organized I am. That day, Donna saw a whole new me.

"What's going on, sweetie?" she asked sweetly.

Instantly, I teared up. "I'm nervous," I blurted. "I don't even know what to wear for cancer treatments."

"Oh, honey, I don't think anyone will be paying attention to your clothes," Donna uttered in the tone of a sweet Care Bear. "It's all about getting you better, not what you look like."

I was in such disarray it felt like I'd never be able to get ready, but Donna quickly got me together. While Donna was helping me, my brother called, and I heard Donna telling him how terrified I was. I don't know what his response was, but two hours later, we arrived in Queens.

Things weren't much better there. My brother had the cold caps and ice…but had gotten too much. Now, he was scrambling to figure out where to store the rest in case we needed more the next day. Dry ice is only good for 24 hours, so the leftovers would go to waste. After much manipulation and finding a second cooler, he was the proud big brother, having completed his part. Next, we loaded the cold caps and our travel bags in the car. Around 8 p.m., the mood was jovial, and we were ready to head out. The atmosphere became tense as we prepared to leave. Everyone seemed wired, including our family dog, Max. My nephews had us laughing as usual, breaking the tension. But the inevitable was upon us; it was time to go.

It was after 11 p.m. when we got to Philly. As soon as we checked into the hotel, Kerry and Loretta dipped out to the casino. I swear, the only reason folks were alright with going to Philly was because it was close to a casino. I don't know what time they got in, but everyone was up and ready for the next day's appointments on time.

Because I was considered a *distant patient* and couldn't come into CTCA the day prior to my appointment for blood work, there was a series of tasks I had to complete before starting my chemo session. I had my blood drawn, had to wait for the doctors to review the results, then be ushered around to another stream of doctors to report how I felt and what effects I'd been feeling from past treatments and prescriptions.

Normally, all of the above would amount to a three to four-hour process, then I'd eat a light lunch and head to the 5th-floor infusion room to be hooked up. But on my first day, I had a discussion with my doctor regarding collapsed veins. Although my veins were good, we had to find the veins and discuss what could happen to them throughout the life of cancer treatments. Without hesitation, I requested a port be inserted inside my chest. I didn't like needles and had been bruised by a nurse who either couldn't find my vein or was just having a bad day. There was no way I was going to let that happen again! The port would ensure less issues, especially in starting and completing the blood-drawing process. It was an unexpected twist in my story, but that day, I had the port inserted. I even recall laughing on the operating table, then waking up with a port in my chest, still laughing.

All of my other appointments (such as chiropractic adjustment and massages) were done while my trio texted, read, relaxed, watched TV, or slept. Finally, I was ready for the infusion. At least, I thought I was. I went to my last appointment with the medical oncologist for her to review my blood work. Well, not only did I have the sniffles, my white blood count (WBC) was low, as it has always been. The two issues were the perfect storm to halt the process. When they told me I couldn't receive my chemo treatment that day, I began sobbing. I felt defeated for a number of reasons.

1. I wanted to start chemo and get it over with.

2. There were a host of people with me, all who had jobs they took off to come with me all the way to Philly, and here we had a false start.

3. Not only had our time been wasted, our money was wasted, too. Yes, money. Not to mention time off work, the time and expense of traveling across two states, and let's not forget the chemo caps that were waiting to be used were rented by the month, and the threat of the dry ice eventually evaporating. All of it, wasted.

Of course, my people didn't blame me. Actually, they were great about everything. We chalked it up to a dry run, even though we were all highly disappointed that my first treatment was a bust.

Every time I think about this first visit, I feel awful. But I'm frequently reminded that the trip wasn't all for naught. Remember, I had the port inserted in my chest. This port was a blessing to me because not only would it be used for chemotherapy but also for blood work. I hated needles so much, I celebrated! However, in full transparency, let me tell you the port was uncomfortable at first. I knew it was there, and my body knew it was foreign.

The first few nights back home after having the port procedure, I couldn't sleep. Suddenly, one day it was causing me severe chest pains, and I couldn't breathe. My mate raced me to the emergency room but had to leave for work. My sorority sister and close friend Monique came to stay with me until my brother arrived. The doctors explained that I was to avoid sleeping on the port, which as a stomach sleeper, felt impossible. They cleared me to go home, and I was released.

Despite the initial discomfort, getting the port was one of the best decisions for me. No matter what center I went to, the first thing they did was draw my blood. With the threat of lymphedema developing in the arm where my lymph nodes were removed, blood was not to be drawn from that arm. Having the port alleviated blood draws solely from my left arm.

The circumstances surrounding not getting the chemo treatment on the first try taught me a lot about myself and my tribe. Everyone became aware of my chronically low white blood count, and I started Neulester before chemotherapy and every visit thereafter. Neulester is a brand name for Neupogen, an injection used to raise the white blood count. This is important because chemotherapy is prone to lower the WBC, making patients more susceptible to infections. With the help of Neulester, I never had an issue with my WBC again and was able to get through all six rounds of chemo treatments. Two weeks after the dry run, we returned, and I successfully had my first treatment thanks to Neulester.

ONE TIRED DAY

One of the side effects of chemotherapy and radiation therapy is fatigue. Although considered one of the lesser side effects, the fatigue you experience is no joke. After the first dose of my chemotherapy regimen, I was physically and mentally out of it; tired was an understatement.

Going into my body, the medicine felt fine. Benadryl helped calm me, but when we finally got back to Queens the next night, I was so tired, and out of it I could cry! This was before we had the system down pat. I wasn't recuperating at Mom's yet and was traveling back to my place in the Bronx.

Mentally, I slipped into a downward spiral. I didn't want to move my car, drive, or even carry my bags in the house when I got home. All I wanted to do was curl up and cry on the sidewalk and lay there for the night. I ended up sitting in the car, weeping. I needed a whole pep talk to get out of the headspace I was in.

On a regular day, my friends have said visiting me is a chore because finding parking where I live is the worst. However, on this particular occasion, it really shouldn't have been that big of a deal because my spot was secured. Donna drove my car from Queens to my house in the Bronx, where she picked up her car and headed home. All I had to do was park my car in the spot she had vacated. That alone seemingly was a huge undertaking. I say this to show how drained I truly was; I literally just wanted to sleep. On the next trip, we switched the process up. Either we both drove, or Donna drove, and I'd work out getting home later. I just didn't want to put myself through driving home after returning from CTCA again.

Reflecting on my journey, the lyrics to the song by gospel duo, Mary Mary ring in my mind: *"Nobody told me the road would be easy, but I don't believe He brought me this far to leave me."* You may find it odd for me to say that this time was one of the hardest points of my journey, but it was the beginning of my treatments, and I felt like I couldn't go on. Like I couldn't carry myself to the next step. Imagine feeling defeated, and you haven't gotten to the super hard stuff yet.

From October 2016 up until now, every day isn't easy, nor is every day hard. A friend once told me that only dead people have nothing to worry about. Living means we'll always face trouble and have concerns; when troubles do rise, I take a step back from the situation and take a few deep breaths. This helps to gain composure, move forward and handle whatever's coming at me. I believe it will help you, too.

I choose to reflect on my cancer journey as a positive because it taught me so much. I still fall back into my old ways at times, eating bad, taking the occasional drink, staying up late, and working long hours. I say *yes* to things I don't like or don't want to do; however, my resilience–my *bounce back* ability, is strong. It's important for me to not only hear my body when it speaks to me, but I listen and do something about it. I try not to stay in a rut too long.

I also recognize when it's time to realign and focus on myself a lot faster. For example, I give my all at work because I want anything attached to my name to be right, and I do what's best for my clients. This leads to a good rating, with better pay. I do my best, but there's only so much one person can do. Everyone won't be happy with everything I do; however, the one thing we must remember is to keep ourselves happy more than 95% of the time. In my book, anything less is unhealthy.

At some point, after I've given all I can or my body and subconscious will allow, I retreat, go deep inward, and bounce back. That's what I did on this particular day. I knew I couldn't lie in the street; as hard as it was, I got myself together and pushed past my feelings. In general, I avoid putting myself in impossible situations where I'll be unhappy. *Do an about-face.* To protect myself and my sanity, my *Yeses* slowly turned to *Nos*. I shorten my work days and even walk slower when I feel like it. (I'm a New Yorker–we do everything fast!).

I've made all these changes, so I may actually feel the sunshine, smell the fresh air and watch the children play. Don't condemn yourself to death! And don't set yourself up for regrets, no matter how big or small, like skipping the massage you really want or something you really feel you should've done. Either you do it, or you don't, but don't beat yourself up with *I should've*. I live in the moment as best I can, doing everything I crave for my peace. It's the little things, like cleaning out the refrigerator, buying fresh fruits and vegetables, and cooking healthy meals when I can. I'm not sure I'll ever be the person to get it done correctly 100% of the time, but I keep striving for better; moving in that direction for me is pure nirvana.

Tell yourself *I love you* when you stick to the commitments you promised yourself. Your inner self (including the child inside) can only learn to trust and love you back when you mean what you say by keeping your word. It's sad to say I spent half my life unaware of the damage I'd done to my reputation with myself. *Lesson learned.* If you don't gain anything else from reading this book, I pray you'll follow through on all the commitments that you make to yourself.

This book is a commitment to myself. My cancer journey is the wake-up call I needed to appreciate the people in my life, especially the ones who agreed to navigate this journey with me. They didn't have to, but they stuck to their "*yes.*" Now while I allow myself all the *Nos* I need, I stick to my commitments to others, unless it's a detriment to myself. And you should, too. Leaving someone high and dry after agreeing to something they've asked you to do is inconsiderate. As long as you're able, finish what you start for yourself and others. If you say yes, do the damn thing because a lackadaisical *yes* sucks.

IT'S GETTING HOT IN HERE

~~~

I knew exactly when I started menopause. Because of the drugs I was taking, I was going to lose my hair and my period. (I was only partially happy with one of those scenarios). Listen, I was happy not to have to worry about blood seeping from my body, bleeding through my jeans onto a chair that I was sitting in, or waking up to soiled bedding from a bloody accident. On the flip side, there were the hot flashes to deal with, which were hell. One doesn't happen because of the other, or vice versa. These are just some of the symptoms of menopause.

I was 41 when my period stopped; it took a year for me to come to grips that it was gone. In April of 2018, I had a *Period END Party*. A couple of friends and I went to a swanky movie theater and celebrated. I gave away the many boxes of pads and panty liners I had accumulated to family, friends, my sorority sisters, and my goddaughter. It didn't take long for me to realize I'd jumped the gun; I was pissed when

I started spotting off and on and had to repurchase a few of the feminine products.

The first two strong hot flashes I had induced the most trauma. My Mom and I talked about menopause, but she never experienced hot flashes, so I wasn't keenly aware of the effects. My eight sisters also didn't give me much insight into the condition. I am, however, in a sorority with virtually hundreds of other women, so I've heard bits and pieces. I've even witnessed women turn red with the rush of heat, but it was hard to picture myself going through it.

One day, while at the gym on the treadmill running at 4.0 up a small hill, I was suddenly paralyzed by heat. I was scorching and thought I was going to pass out! I got a little scared, stopped running, and gulped some water, but then went on without thinking anything of it. I left the gym and didn't mention what happened to anyone. If the flashes weren't consistent, there was no need to worry anyone about it.

The next flash struck while I was on Amtrak heading home from CTCA. I had just completed a treatment, it was the dead of the winter, and Donna and I were bundled up next to the door that kept opening and closing at every stop, letting the chilly air inside. All at once, that rush of heat came over me, and I immediately stripped my top layer of clothes–coat, hat, scarf, sweater; next thing Donna turned around, and I took my shirt off. I was down to my camisole, still hot but much better. Donna, in her Care Bear voice, asked, "Uhm, are you okay?" I muttered "Yes", and we both burst out laughing. It was after that episode that I spoke to my doctors about the hot flashes I was experiencing. The naturopath suggested the homeopathic medicine–Acteane, which was hormone free and would help relieve hot flashes.

Months later, I was so used to hot flashes that I wasn't paying them much attention anymore. I just went through the motions and moved on. The issue was I had a flash to hit after my breast radiation treatment; the heat that hit me was unlike any other time I'd ever experienced before. It was maybe a week or two after radiation therapy had been completed, and I'd gone to Las Vegas on the trip that I had been planning for months. I jumped through hurdles just to take this trip.

I was able to save my hair, but it wasn't the texture I expected. My hair was dry and brittle and lacked fullness and density, so different than I wanted or anticipated. As a result, I braided it up and wore a wig. I was menopausal, having hot flashes, fresh off the heels of radiation, trapped in a wig, and subjected to the desert heat…all recipes for disaster!

During one of our national sorority conventions, there were thousands of women and men in town. We were edged out of most hotels (including the host hotel) but lucked out with a place to stay at my sorority sister's timeshare not far from Las Vegas Blvd. From the hotel, we took the hotel shuttle, walked or caught an Uber. With the crowds of people in town, there was a delay in most modes of transportation, except for good ole walking. Uber was also new to me and scarce in Vegas. There was a time when we got into an Uber, and the license plate was different from what showed up in my phone. We were desperate but swore off doing it again.

Having some time to kill before my session, I decided to take the shuttle from my hotel to Harrah's Casino since it was my first free moment to play the slots. Instead of waiting for the next bus, I walked a short distance to the Bellagio. The walk is only about half a mile, maybe 10 minutes, which is slow and long when you're in the heat, lugging bags around. All I needed to do was get across to the west side of the Las Vegas boulevard, walk one block south, then up the overpass steps, which crosses over Flamingo Road, and into the air-conditioned building. A third of the way there, I was positive I was going to pass out.

I was so hot and tired, I wanted to curl up on the sidewalk and die (Sidebar: This is my second mention of such a feeling. Cancer fatigue hits different). I couldn't last another moment in the street; I was so exhausted. Trudging on, I finally made it to the building, where I plopped in the lobby and promptly rested in the AC for about 30 minutes without moving. The sorority sisters passing me by asked if I was okay; I wasn't, but I smiled and waved them on. After a while,

I cooled off, gained my composure, and made it to my destination on the other side of the building.

There was a combination of factors that really knocked me out. The Vegas heat, the wig, sheer tiredness—which is a side effect of radiation. I took things very slow during radiation, sleeping in, and limiting the places I drove, since the hotel bus picked us up or the CTCA limo picked me up daily.

Making the trip to Vegas, then trying to get back to normal was obviously doing too much. I didn't even let my friends know about the Vegas incident until much later when it was almost funny to tell it. All I wanted was some independence on this trip. If I'd told folks about it, there would've been zero possibility of that actually happening.

Pearl of Wisdom #15: Whether you have flashes due to age or cancer treatments such as chemotherapy and radiation, they come on suddenly without warning. To help prepare yourself, carry a fan and a bottle of water with you. Depending on where you live, the weather and seasons can be tricky, so try dressing in layers that can be removed when the flashes hit. I know it's important to get back to normal and maintain your independence, but it's imperative to keep someone abreast of your whereabouts while you're out having fun. This is for your own well-being.

NATUROPATH

~~~

The multitude of drugs and supplements during my cancer journey included chemotherapy drugs Taxotere (aka, Docetaxel) and Cytoxan (aka, Cyclophosphamide). Wanting to treat the whole body in addition to destroying the cancer, I enlisted two naturopaths. My goal had always been to supplement with naturopathic medicine, as well as holistic treatments for my entire body. Not only did CTCA administer all the traditional treatments, but they also let cancer patients supplement with homeopathic medicine, which was important to me.

While on chemotherapy, I was given iron to prevent iron deficiency and took the following supplements to heal faster following treatments:

- Eupatorium Perfoliatum 30C - Homeopathic supplement used to relieve stiffness and bone pain

- Drosera 30C - Homeopathic supplement used to relieve spasmodic dry cough
- Coq10 - targets energy and vital organ support, heart muscle, and kidneys.
- 81mg of aspirin.
- Melatonin to induce sleep and harvest a healthy immune system; rumored to have anti-cancer properties.
- Vitamin D to support the immune system and bone health.
- Omega 3 coated triglyceride, a form of fish oil which is anti-inflammatory and possibly beneficial in cancer preventative measures.
- Astragalus - immune support and increases white blood cell counts.
- L glutamine powder, which eases neuropathy. Not to be taken with food.
- Zinc, which increases white blood cell counts (as per the internet and Loretta).

I cannot speak on what others took or miracle drugs that I didn't take; I can only speak on what I took and what helped me and boosted my immune system. There's something called the placebo effect, which means there was the possibility that everything I was taking actually did nothing at all, and the improvements were only in my head. Regardless of this fact, I was still all in.

I was supposed to meet with another naturopathic doctor outside of CTCA to obtain Vitamin C intravenously, as well as German Mistletoe, also known as Iscador. However, I never made it to him. Instead, I worked with my specialist at CTCA to start Astragalus, Maitake, and herbal biotics, all of which combatted the chemo, radiation, and surgery side effects while helping to boost my immune system, similar to the effects of Vitamin C infusions and German Mistletoe.

There are many drugs and supplements on the market that are not FDA-approved yet widely and successfully used, some of which I've taken myself. Nothing illegal, but there was one time I ended up in urgent care with my blood levels out of whack, my arm partially swollen, and based on the blood panel taken, no one could figure out what happened to me. Days before, I'd been in the woods, so we assumed maybe I'd gotten a tick bite, with the possibility of Lyme disease setting in. Once that was ruled out, my doctors had me run down the list of everything I was taking, and we determined it was the apricot supplement. After that, I've never ingested the seed, pill, or pit again. The aftermath wasn't worth it.

While I was okay with supplementing without supervision before cancer, I learned the hard way that I probably should not supplement on my own with things I'd read or heard about via the internet during my cancer journey. In this case, I read that apricots were a cure for cancer. I found what I believed was a decent supplement and started taking it. I was careful, read the instructions, took it with food, and followed the directions to the letter. No matter what precautions I took, it wasn't a good experience or supplement for me. Why? Because apricot seeds contain a plant toxin, which can convert to cyanide and be harmful to the body. **(Source: https://www.sciencedirect.com/science/article/abs/pii/S0196064498700770)**

With the exception of this one time, I made my naturopathic doctor aware of everything I was ingesting. Certified naturopathic practitioners who are either in communication with your oncologist or you acting as the liaison is vital. Make sure to advise both doctors what you are taking and how it leaves you feeling. At CTCA, the naturopathic practitioner suggested I avoid harsh prescription medication, substituting them with herbal supplements first. There were other times when the medical oncologist shrugged off the supplements, saying they wouldn't affect or interfere with my treatments.

No matter how anyone felt, I believed I was doing what was right for me and my body, with consultation from the correct people. It's important to be present, alert, and an active, willing participant in your journey. Of course, at first, everything is new and scary, and folks are bombarding you with all sorts of information that can be overwhelming. You should welcome all the help and information you can get, but take ownership of your own health.

I was rarely talked at by my doctors, but when I was, I dismissed them. Of the three centers I have gone to, one thing the cancer doctors have in common is compassion. Some talk too fast or may forget that the patient they're talking to is new to this, but they care, and they listen intently. I never felt as if I wasn't being heard by my core team of doctors. There are things I still want to try to improve my health, such as intravenous Vitamin C. According to *Utopia Cancer Center*, it promotes immune health and can kill cancer cells.

The moral of this story is when you are on chemo and decide to take other supplements, you must be careful, upfront, and vocal about what you're doing on your own, and you must have your blood drawn so that your levels can be monitored for issues that may need immediate tending to. For example, taking garlic prior to surgery or antioxidants (such as basic prenatal pills) shouldn't be taken with chemo regimens as it lowers the effectiveness. **(Source: https://pubmed. ncbi.nlm.nih.gov/17761641/)**

We've all heard about not drinking or eating grapefruit while on various drugs like blood pressure pills. I'm not sure what's in it that dilutes the effects of our regular medications; however, these simple drug interactions can be detrimental to your health.

MY BREASTS AND SEXUALITY

I've only just started to look at my breasts in the mirror again. They are different. One is my age; she looks good as she lies there. She's my muse. She hasn't betrayed me. Then there is the saucy one. She is younger yet more experienced and has been through some trauma. She's outrageous and speaks out for causes. She is still standing and not here for the shit. And while she commands love and attention, she's somewhat meek, tender, and at times doesn't want to be looked at or touched.

Let me clear up what I mean by *betray me.* Yes, there was a time that I felt betrayed by my breast. However, after much-needed heart work between me, myself, and my breasts, instead of thinking my breasts tried to kill me, I feel that my breasts woke me up and saved me. I've never ever hated myself or my body, and definitely not my breasts; it was time to reassure them that I saw, heard, and would protect them for the rest of my life.

Pearl of Wisdom #16: Do mirror work. Look at yourself in the mirror, smile, and love on yourself. Tell yourself it's safe to be who you are, to feel safe in your skin, to love again, and be touched again. Forgive yourself. Try saying this: (Insert your name), I love you, trust you, and will protect you. You did nothing wrong–never can and never will!

I do this while caressing my breasts, truly feeling the energy and love inside of them.

I also had a man wanting to love me during this time. Before I healed from feeling that my breasts betrayed me, I thought that they were ugly. So, it was difficult to let down the walls and let love in. When we're feeling this way, we need to take a step back. I've never been overly sexual or lusting for sex. I wanted it when I wanted it. I pleased my mate well but didn't want to be bothered outside of that. Factor in two post-surgeries, chemotherapy, and radiation, and the last thing I wanted was sex on a regular basis. After my treatments were complete, sex rarely crossed my mind.

There were other factors to be considered as well. Follow me on this, years before the start of this journey, I was rubbing progesterone cream on myself to regulate hormones. A close friend told me that products I introduced myself to were considered transdermal application, could seep into my bloodstream, and rub off on my mate, too. I've since learned better, but still, the thought was amplified. So although I desperately wanted to be held, in a twisted way, I was trying to protect my mate, pushing him away because I didn't want the chemo drugs to rub off on him. (Remember, when I had the procedure, I was told not to hold babies or pets on my chest).

I also heard a conversation while going through chemo and learned that the toilets at CTCA double flushed to keep the fluids from contaminating other patients. And actually, I recall non-patients using a separate bathroom. All of these scenarios were embedded in my mind, none of which were verified by doctors. I didn't want the toxins to rub off on my mate and have his penis develop issues from being exposed to me. Look, I didn't say every thought during my chemo journey was rational.

On top of everything else, I didn't want sex because I didn't feel desirable or sexy. I'm not saying that I needed the lights out during sex, but I also didn't want a light shined on me. My breasts are lopsided because I chose not to do reconstructive surgery. I didn't want to subject myself to any more surgery. Besides, as a cancer patient, you have a lifetime guarantee to go back and have reconstruction.

Finally, let's not forget that following surgery, breast sensations are different, and there's scar tissue left behind. My doctors reconnected what they could, but that area remains tender to this day. Years later, I have odd sensations in my breast. Around the time

I had surgery, I was extremely on edge about laying a certain way for fear of bruising myself. Add a man groping me to the mix, and I wasn't there for any of it. I'm not a hard person to love, but I can recognize when I made it hard to love me.

I eventually got past some of these issues, but then I started feeling obligated to perform. Honestly, I wanted love, to curl up inside a man's arms and rest, but it wasn't in me to perform. I wanted to be left alone. From experience, I can tell you to give yourself grace. You're learning the new version of yourself; there's no going back. As my poem, *Same Difference*, below states, you are new and different. The way you approach life and love before and after cancer are different. In many ways, cancer taught me how to teach others how to love me, how to treat me, and the things I will and won't tolerate.

Sex, breasts and healthy relationships are integral to the journey. You get to decide how it looks, who gets to touch you, and who gets to experience the joy and energy that you have inside to give. Remember, you are going through treatment–the little you have to give should be spent on you first and foremost and the most special people and things in your life, secondly.

Same Difference

A voice in my head asks, who are you?

It asks, where are you?

It states, you are unrecognizable!

I reply: I am me, I am here staring at you in the mirror, I am the same person I've always been!

The voice states, not sure you have noticed, but somewhere between always and today, things have changed.

As I begin to utter, what do you mean......

A list is rattled off

Your smile is different

Personality different

Hair wayyy different

Skin different

Nails different

Sleep pattern different

Energy level different

Tolerance different

Family bonds different

Friendships different

Needs, wants and desires all different

Stamina different

My breasts are different

You are wholesale regarded differently.

I wonder in my head, nothing is the same, nothing will ever be the same. A piece of me is missing, I am no longer whole or complete. I am fragments of the whole. I am 1-in-8.

I tried so hard to remain the same that, be it good or bad,
I stopped noticing the differences.

I blurt out, sameness is overrated, so you can stop looking for me like a stalker in the night.

My perfectly old norm is gone, my new norm stands before you, ready for the world.

UGLY DUCKLING

I am a regular, around-the-way girl who's had both good days and bad days. Some of my darkest days came after the first surgery I had. Let me reiterate that you cannot manage cancer; cancer came out of nowhere, but I had plans that I refused to miss. I wasn't the only one I knew who turned 40 in 2016. A few close friends and family members of mine did as well, and we had big plans!

At the top of that year, I started out strong, celebrating my birthday in Barbados. Then in July, I went to Europe, and in December, I was heading back to Barbados to celebrate Donna's birthday. From the time I learned of my diagnosis, I started intentionally managing my doctors appointments so I'd be in the best position to celebrate in Barbados with my girls. I was happy to be physically able to take the trip, but someone should've warned me that I'd be slammed with mental challenges. After surgery and on that Barbados trip, I felt so ugly.

Most women will tell you when we get ready for a trip or even a simple day out with friends, you have to show up correct. Hair done, nails done, everything done. Unfortunately, I couldn't pull it together. I was physically worn out and unable to complete all of my pre-trip activities, like getting my hair braided so I wouldn't have to worry about my hair on a tropical island.

So, here's the thing: I did not feel like sitting for hours to get long, elaborate braids, so I settled for a simple pattern that I hated. The style I got made my head look big, but it was better than wasting precious time in the hair salon. I basically fell out of surgery and rolled onto a plane, then headed straight for the beach when I landed. I was delighted to be there but wasn't mentally prepared for how I'd feel around people. For the most part, everyone was apprised of my situation, but still, I felt uneasy. This trip wasn't about me, so I faked being okay to avoid appearing needy or weak.

I was in the company of more than 20 other beautiful women of all shapes, sizes, and colors who unknowingly made me feel very inadequate because I felt I lacked sex appeal. I couldn't shake the fact that someone had just gone in and altered my body. My scar was healing but far from appealing. At this point, I was at odds with my body, curious about why it allowed all of these horrible things to happen to *us*. The word betrayed was still being tossed around in my head. I've never been overweight, but had gotten so shockingly skinny. I was forced to wear compression tops all day, so I fashioned the ones from Victoria's Secret into swimwear, but it paled in comparison to what the other women were wearing on this trip. Every bathing suit I saw was more colorful and prettier than the last. I hated everything about my look and style. I felt like an ugly duckling who'd never be beautiful again.

I shunned special treatment, but I did crave compassion. Whether it was true or not, I even felt like my roommate didn't give me leeway or sympathy. On one hand, I desperately wanted to be and feel normal, but I wasn't. To the world, I was 100% back to myself; little did they know I was operating off 50% and didn't want folks treating me as if I was completely restored.

Despite my misgivings, the trip was good for many reasons. As we celebrated life, I kept telling myself that life goes on. The surgery was a little more than two weeks before the trip. My life was forever changed. While other patients would opt to stay home, there I was, gallivanting in another country.

My friend had a cousin who made everyone feel seen and had us laughing and smiling for hours. On every Barbados trip, he catered to us, but since he knew what was going on with me, he was extra attentive. See, he had a way of making folks feel good about life and everything coming on the horizon. He was just that type of island guy. On this particular trip, he secured transportation for the entire group at the airport but had me ride with him to avoid bumpy roads that would be harmful to me post-surgery. He was a gem to me the entire trip and paid me extra attention that I wasn't aware I needed at that moment but that I deserved and graciously accepted.

The trip allowed me to appreciate the good things in life. Barbados is beautiful! We sat at the beach, drank, went on excursions, took pictures, shared laughs, and reminisced. I thoroughly needed that time away to do exactly what I've been encouraging you to do throughout this book: Keep living, keep doing, keep thriving, and keep getting up…even as you fight cancer! I refused to let cancer keep me down. I enjoyed myself whether cancer wanted me to or not; the only drawback during my time away was that while I was determined to keep moving and living, I wasn't as spry as I usually was. The group didn't say anything, but I believe *the new me* made some of them uncomfortable. Hell, I was even a little upset with myself.

My roommate finally had enough and dealt me some serious tough love. "You're not sick anymore," she said. "You had surgery already; let's go!"

One thing you should know is that I'm always slow. Whenever we traveled to sorority conferences, the hotel rooms were always packed, and bathroom time was limited. All of my roommates know that I'm usually first in the bathroom because I need a jump start on everyone else. Even with the extra time, I still wind up being last out of our room.

While we were in Barbados, I felt left behind a couple of times, and it hurt. When I needed care the most, it was lacking from my friend. Thankfully, we've since talked about and gotten far past that point. What I hadn't considered was that she was just as afraid and uncomfortable as I was. Having a friend going through cancer surgery and treatment is not something everyone in life has dealt with or was equipped for. And I got it wrong a couple of times myself. I failed to express what I needed at the time, so I got what people gave me. I can't fault others for that.

Pearl of Wisdom #17: As cancer patients, it's imperative to express your feelings to those in your close circle. Tell them how you feel and what you need. It doesn't have to be a big, long, drawn-out discussion. However, in order to be supported the way you need and desire, you have to open up about your needs, as well as what does and doesn't work for you. Given my strong, independent background, cancer was an extremely vulnerable journey to embark upon.

RADIATION

Radiation was an oddly fun time for me. I chose to do it right before the start of summer. I opted to use my Family Medical Leave to take time off from work. I spent three weeks in Philadelphia, including the Fourth of July weekend. I met new friends, reacquainted with old friends, enjoyed a free concert, and stayed in a beautiful apartment complex in downtown Philly that one of my sorority sisters connected me to. I fit in some sightseeing, too.

I always kept in the back of my mind that although the cancer was gone after the surgeries and chemotherapy I had, radiation was necessary to ensure there was nothing microscopic left in the breast. Day one of radiation was scary but magical. This was something I'd have to do over the course of a few weeks, so I quickly adjusted. My brother was with me the first couple of days; however, no one could be there with me every day. Still, I knew I had support.

Now on the third day of treatment, I was on the CTCA bus, headed from the hotel to the center. It was like the first day of school, riding the bus alone, except I was 41 and had an iPhone, taking pictures of myself on the way. I spoke to Kerry, Donna, and Mom that morning and every day while I was there. They knew so much about the layout of the land; they called or texted, asked if I was eating, back at the hotel, or what did *Dr. So-and-So* say (calling them by name). Even without my support team physically present, they were always there for me.

Toward the end, I did have second thoughts about choosing CTCA. Had I been in NYC, I could probably have someone with me every day, but then I'd be denying myself all the services CTCA had under a single roof. And not having to drive myself took a load of the pressure off. It was painless and seamless; that's what I desired most.

The radiation room I was in was huge. You walked down the hall, turned left, and it's like you landed in a park or something. It was breezy in there, but then again, it could've been the hospital gown, leggings, and flip-flops I was wearing.

Facing you as you walk in, there's a huge, electronic, gorgeous mural sprawled across the wall. So stunning; it was more like a painting. My radiologist was laid back and easy with me. With others, I'm sure he had a lot more work to do, but by the time I came to him, my case was rather simple. During my last surgery, he worked with the breast surgeon, and I had Intraoperative Radiation Therapy (IORT) which was a single high-dose boost of targeted radiation. Doctors said I still needed external beam radiation after the IORT, so I went along with it. Most of my time was spent with the radiology techs–the nicest Black female and a Black male who was her sidekick. Together, they were like a comedy show, asking me what music I wanted to hear and blasting it in the room. My answer was always the same: Mary J. Blige. So, they stopped asking and played her music for me during every visit.

Radiation lasted no more than 25 minutes. It took longer to get undressed and wait for one of the rooms to be reconfigured from the patient who was seen before me. The treatment itself wasn't the worst thing ever, but it was uncomfortable. You must lay in a certain position, and stop moving and breathing upon command. Afterward, I was always stiff! It was hard lying in an odd position for that long; it felt like my blood drained out.

Radiation was my time of reflection. Of my entire cancer journey, I think this was the time I enjoyed the most. It was close to the end of the process, and I took off work as my doctors recommended. It was three weeks of being in my skin. This was really *me time*; while I had learned to be pretty selfish with my time during my journey, this was when I dug in even deeper. Cancer is scary, but it's important to honor it and understand why things occurred to prevent repeating them.

Admittedly, I got down to some of those levels I didn't need to be on. Not having people around allowed me time to hear my own thoughts and tend to my feelings without interruption. I wasn't working, and my people weren't with me. This time was needed, but I felt alone for the first time during my journey. Dr. Allie instructed me to meditate, do yoga, and journal to understand my feelings and cope with the loneliness and fears I had.

I wound up replacing journaling and meditating every day with an introspective journey outside of my normal habits. Daily, I woke up and did some type of movement. Once the winter weather warmed up, I was able to walk CTCA's garden and walking path. Then back at the hotel, I hopped in the pool for exercise, followed by perusing the stores on Roosevelt Boulevard. I've never been a napper, but I napped, too. I wasn't tired, but I'd gone on a retreat to Block Island once before, and the owner of the bread and breakfast where I stayed explained there weren't televisions in the guest room, so our brains could rest. I took a queue from that trip and took naps during the day to allow my brain to rest.

I walked downtown Philadelphia for miles, strolled through Love Park, window-shopped, visited the observation deck of One Liberty Place, lounged at the street fairs, and admired the water fountains. This point in time was unlike any other in my life.

The radiation treatments were a great time of self-reflection for me. Going out on FMLA helped me to do that. I was only scratching the surface, but it was a good start. Technically if I worked during chemo, I could've worked during radiation. But by then, my mindset had shifted. At the start of my journey, I was scared of losing my job. Work helped me focus on other things besides cancer. By late 2017, I was ready to lose the superwoman cape. People think Black women are so strong and fearless that we can tolerate more pain. Extreme pain. In some respects, I can understand why people feel that way, but it's largely untrue.

While we are strong, Black women get tired, feel uncomfortable, have been hurt, want to be held, and don't want to always be seen as breadwinners. We are treasures who want to be cherished. If my job was going to make up something to fire me when I returned from leave, then so be it! It obviously wasn't meant to be. It was more important for me to honor my health and my body by not working during radiation. I viewed the radiation treatments differently than chemotherapy, though they served the same purpose. Radiation was more of a retreat, a time of building myself back up and becoming stronger.

I didn't excuse myself from the office to do more; I took off to do less. This was my time to rebuild. Of course, there was more time to do other things. Since I wasn't at home cleaning my house or doing my laundry list of never-ending tasks…I was simply enjoying life.

Considering that a three-week hotel stay would be too much, I stayed at a friend of a friend's house for my first week of radiation. Her house was less than 10 minutes from the 30th Street Station, so I made arrangements to leave my car at CTCA and be picked up by the car service.

I thoroughly enjoyed the independence I had, staying outside of CTCA. Folks on the outside had no idea you had cancer, which helped give me the normalcy I was missing. To them, I was just another tourist. I spent many days walking the streets, exploring my surroundings in the summer heat.

I'm not the best cook, but I was cooking up cuisines like I was a top chef. There was something about shopping at Trader Joe's grocery store that I loved. I never shop there, but I was enjoying being an entirely new me. When I didn't cook, I tried some of the restaurants I'd heard about in town. At night, I lay on my friend's couch with the shades draped over the large bay windows open, so the city lights could shine in. I also volunteered at one of the oldest known African-American-owned plots in Philly– Mother Bethel AME Church in City Center. This was a pit stop along the Underground Railroad. This time I spent at the friend's home felt like a low-key vacation.

The remainder of my two-week stay was mostly spent at the Four Points Sheraton near CTCA. One of the many shining spots during my stay was connecting with my college roommate, Natasha. She and I have been friends for over 20 years; we speak a few times a year to catch up. I left my cancer center on a Friday after treatment and drove northeast to see her. It was so much fun to finally be able to visit and spend time in her world. I've always loved Natasha, even when our communication dwindled to speaking on birthdays, holidays, or the occasional visit. Funny how life changes. Now I had cancer, and Natasha had a husband and a baby boy she was preparing a first birthday party for.

For the party, Natasha had set up a bouncy house and water slide, both of which I played on like a big kid, and had a blast! Arriving in Delaware was surreal. Seeing Natasha after all those years, grown up and married, was mind-blowing. All I could think about was the night she graduated the year after me, and the limo ride to the celebration. It was a night to be remembered.

Memories like that bring me back to my youth and the fun times we had. I wanted more of that. For the party, I jumped right in, helping Natasha prepare the house. We laughed hard about everything all night. The next day, it was pure joy seeing Natasha celebrate her love and life with family and loved ones. That Sunday, we slowed the pace. Natasha, her cousin, and I walked through her neighborhood. They asked me about how my journey was going, and I filled them in. We laughed, cried, and enjoyed the soul food we were feeding each other's spirits. It was a time I won't forget.

That Monday, I headed back to Philadelphia for my final week of radiation. I was back at the hotel, and Donna joined me for my final days. The Independence Day celebration was upon us, and Philadelphia was alive! I'd seen that my favorite artist–Mary J. Blige, was headlining Philly's annual 4th celebration. I was determined to get out there and be in the mix! On a regular day, Philadelphia is alive with love and culture. It's the City of Brotherly Love, after all. Both the Declaration of Independence and the United States Constitution were written in Philadelphia, so naturally, some refer to Philly as the birthplace of America, making it a force to be reckoned with come Independence Day!

Since it was a holiday, CTCA was closed. No radiation treatment, but also no cars to take us into Philly. Fortunately, the hotel's concierge helped map the way for us to use public transportation. We took a bus (which turned into a cable car-bus-train combination), then hopped on the real train, which took us to Market Street, where we perused the attractions.

We finally made it to the mecca of fun, which was close to the Philadelphia Museum of Art…featuring the steps featured in the *Rocky* movie. The street fair was already in progress, so we walked around, shopped, ate, and waited for the concert to begin. It was a sunny, warm day, with not a cloud in sight. Having arrived so early, I started to tire out, but there was no chance we were leaving before the big show.

To kill time, Donna and I sat around, talking and people-watching. We weren't close to the stage, but at least we were in the atmosphere. Everything was great until it started raining. People scattered, but I stayed right where I was, shielded by my trusty umbrella. The good thing was we were able to move close to the stage and grab a couple of seats. It seemed like hours passed before the show began after sunset. City officials gave greetings, and Boys II Men opened up. I had never seen them in concert, so that was a rare treat. When Mary J. Blige took the stage, I couldn't believe how up close and personal we were to witness her live in concert, absolutely free! It was so nice. MJB is one of my favorite artists; her music is the soundtrack of my life. No matter what I'm going through, there's always a song to fit my mood…which is always elevated by music.

After the concert, there was a fireworks display in the distance. We enjoyed the show, then took the reverse ride home, train to bus. It was a bit scarier at night, but Donna and I made it back in one piece.

My radiation journey helped sustain my health. It wrapped up the entire process with a bow and sealed it with a kiss. I was confident that cancer was gone for good.

THERAPY

~~~

I would be lying if I said that I breezed through my cancer journey and treatments because I absolutely didn't.

You have cancer.

After hearing those words, I cried for three days straight. The tears suddenly stopped, and I was ready to fight. For the rest of my journey, I didn't cry. At least not outright. I would tear up or fall into a tantrum, but crying wasn't an option. Over the course of my life, I've been conditioned to think that crying is a sign of weakness or guilt. I internalized everything people told me and sequestered my emotions because of what they said. My heart is on my sleeve, and there is no mistaking how I feel by looking at my face. But I refused to allow my tears to tell the story.

Between working out, being active in my sorority and the NPHC, and helping my friend through her mother's critical illness, I piled too much on my plate. I can see now that it was a coping mechanism. Not that it was at the forefront of my mind when I started my cancer journey, but I knew about the benefits of mental health therapy early on. Even before being diagnosed, I'd seen multiple therapists.

A few weeks into chemotherapy, I spotted a therapy session on my schedule but didn't think much of it. The first few sessions were filled with fluff, and I didn't think it was a great fit for me. For months, I did what I could to dodge those appointments. It wasn't until almost two years out of active treatment that things started getting real. We talked about my sleepless nights, excessive crying, and out-of-control emotions. Finally, my therapist pinpointed what I was dealing with, PTSD. PTSD (*Post Traumatic Stress Disorder*) is an anxiety disorder that can result from a shocking, scary, or dangerous event. **Source: (https://www.nimh.nih. gov/health/topics/post-traumatic-stress-disorder-pts- d#part3)**

It wasn't until we talked meds that I really started listening. One of my sisters suffers from mental illness and refuses to consistently take her medication. I'd always told myself that if I faced taking medication for anything, I'd do it to improve my quality of life. Welp, here I was, faced with that very decision. A year later, I made the choice.

I recall that my cherished GYN explained that I should do *talk therapy* before considering medications. On one hand, I was told not to take medication; on the other, I was told talk therapy takes too long, so I needed the pills. Either way, I felt hopeless.

Allow me to dissect this a bit more, as this topic is one of the most important in this book.

While I was open to taking medication, meeting with the psychiatrist at the center wasn't helpful at first. Perhaps because I was afraid. I sat quietly while she talked about her kids and her dogs. It was nice because she was colorful and animated. The sessions were pleasant enough–no pressure or discomfort. I swear, after our sessions, I felt better about my life, but that's because we never dug past the surface. It wasn't the therapist's fault, though. I wasn't being open and vulnerable like I should've been. In the past, I'd been to therapy, all with older white women. All of them were kind, even the one who closed her eyes and seemingly fell asleep during one of our sessions.

Talk therapy was okay, but I really wasn't getting the full benefit from it. Still, I forged on, telling the psychiatrist I didn't want medication. All was fine until suddenly, I was going to CTCA alone, no more fun family rides, my childhood home was being sold, Mom was moving, and I was sad and depressed and battling PTSD.

I was present throughout my cancer journey while simultaneously on autopilot. I did whatever I could just to get past all of it. In 2018, I began feeling the brunt of the surgeries, chemo, and radiation. Everything I'd gone through hit me like a ton of bricks. I was sad, weepy, and unable to sleep. Anger rose within me. The biggest trigger for me was the **For Sale** sign in the front yard. Mom was moving away; my childhood home was gone. "But what if the cancer comes back?" I asked. "I guess it can't because there's no house to convalesce in!" No home. No peace. Not even a mother in the same state to help if things fell apart.

I needed to find someone that I could work with because the assigned psychiatrist at CTCA was too far, and I needed consistent appointments. I knew I could not go back to the person that closed her eyes during one of my sessions, so I searched the doctors that took my insurance. As an insurance pick, I wasn't expecting much, but my first choice was Shirley Taylor Dunn, who had two things going for her: she's a woman, and her office is close to my home. As a bonus, when I contacted her, I could tell she was Black. Our first visit was what set my heart on fire. The doctor was extremely direct, in your face, and no-nonsense. She even resembled a dark-skinned version of my Aunt Eileen, who is all cheekbone, and whom I love dearly. And like Aunt Eileen, Shirley commanded attention.

Mrs. Dunn got me straight. She helped me understand why the meds may be beneficial to me. Outside of being a Pisces, she noted that I seemed overly weepy and downtrodden. I was actually following in the footsteps of the very thing I'd worked to avoid. But a part of me felt like taking medication was almost a "requirement" to see her. I soon realized though, that by no means was she forcing meds on me, but she simply wanted to see me progress past where I was. Over a month after first meeting her and seeing the psychiatrist at CTCA (sometimes you need both), I started taking Lexapro, which is used to treat depression and anxiety.

Lexapro improved my mood, but that didn't stop me from counting the days until I was able to get off of it. I wound up staying on those pills through most of the pandemic; they actually helped usher me through 2020. But the holistic side of me knew the toxicity and multiple side effects medication can bring on, not to mention the weight gain I experienced. I'm not completely sure if the pounds I packed on was pandemic or medication weight, but two years later, I'm still fighting to reduce the almost 20-30 pound increase after starting the medication.

Now in late 2021 (as I'm writing this book), I realize that I probably still needed Lexapro as the pandemic raged on. However, in early 2021, everything came to a screeching halt. I stopped taking meds, I stopped seeing the therapist, Mom moved, my brother wasn't there, and friends and relationships were crumbling. Everything that had held me together for so long was gone. My friend, Donna, who helped me, was now off tending to her own life, and our relationship was strained for many reasons. I felt so alone.

I've since started back to therapy weekly; sometimes I take a few weeks off, but therapy will remain a part of my life for the rest of my life.

Pearl of Wisdom #18: I recommend therapy for everyone; it's nothing to be ashamed of. Talking to a third party who isn't part of your family or circle of friends is beneficial, especially when battling a deadly disease. A therapist can help you see and address things differently, and they're more objective.

My therapist always sees situations from an angle that I may not have considered. She challenges me to think outside of the box while presenting me with ways I could've handled things differently. She also reels me back in when I spiral out or worry whether the cancer is returning. In addition to my treatments, my therapist helped save my life. Talk therapy works.

ENDINGS

～～～

Life will never be the same. Many things had to end or terminate for me to understand that. Since being out of active treatment, so many things ended or were removed from my life that I was baffled by it all. That means God was using them to speak to me.

There's no going back, though; we can only move forward. What was most important to remember was that CANCER also ended. I had everything I needed, a home to recuperate in, nearby family to take care of me, doctors who'd drop everything and return my calls, and access to the best medical facility on planet Earth. I had built-in help and love–the best weapons to fight cancer!

By mid 2018, I had completed my year of treatments. I remember how I cried because I wanted to get started with chemotherapy and finish so I could get on with the rest of the procedures I needed to heal. Once I was out of that stage, I felt far from finished. I was still visiting CTCA every couple of months...completely oblivious to what was coming that would soon shake me to the core.

The selling of my childhood home and over 30 years' worth of memories, along with it, set off the chain of events. Selfishly I thought, *What about me?* That house was the gathering spot, the core of our lives. We gathered there to strategize and prepare before heading to Philly; it's where I recouped after treatment and got nursed back to health. Every birthday, holiday, prom, and graduation all started and ended at that house. Since I didn't move until I was 32, the house saw its fair share of my live-in boyfriends too. I even lost my virginity between those walls! Our home was a pit stop for everyone flying in or out of Laguardia Airport. I hadn't lived there in many years, but it was still my go-to place.

Selling the house was like losing a friend. I've never experienced mourning the death of an inanimate object, but I quickly found out that it was a thing. From my perspective, the house had seen approximately five generations walk through its doors. In its heyday (before some conversions), it was a 4-story, 8-bedroom, 2-bath house with two kitchens and a 2-car garage that could fit five cars in the driveway. After the conversions, the basement was finished, and we added two additional bathrooms. Our house, along with a few other houses on the block, threw show-stopping barbecues that folks talked about long after the party was over.

So many good things happened there, but in the end, the house was unfortunately too old and drained too much money. Despite this, I seriously considered purchasing it and my ex-boyfriend even priced its value. It was too much house for me. I was furious with the decision to sell, but I also had no leg to stand on. Once that **For Sale** sign went up in the front yard, I knew it was the beginning of the end.

Selling the house contributed to my need for therapy. Mom was 73 years old when my brother settled on selling the house, and Mom decided to move over 300 miles away, which would require a nearly seven-hour drive to see her. I swelled with pride, seeing Mom stand up for herself and do what was best for her own well-being, but my goodness, this was a severe blow to me! I may have been grown, living on my own, but I was very much a cancer patient going through the motions. Honestly, I was devastated to "lose" Mom. Sometimes for no reason at all, I showed up at the house, and she'd move the tons of magazines and newspapers from beside her, then I curled up next to her and went to sleep. I wasn't sure how I'd make it without Mom. Even at the printing of this book, it's still one of the things I struggle with most in life–not having my mother close to me.

Selling the house meant my family was disbanded. It was traumatic, but having my immediate family scattered is what threw me over the top. My nephews disappeared from my life for a while, but my brother ended up being super close to me for a time. We lived five minutes from each other in the Bronx. It was great to have him nearby.

During the pandemic, my brother retired and eventually moved over 1000 miles away from me. All of these life *endings* were starting to take a toll on me. All I could think about was what if the pandemic never ends, and I can't travel to see my mother or brother. My therapist frequently reminded me that they're both alive and while no one was sure what would come of the pandemic, I could call or video chat with them. I preferred in-person communication as opposed to a concept that was foreign to me; however, I had to get used to it…nothing would ever be the same from here on out.

All of these *endings* hit in a span of mere months. And they kept coming. One day my dermatologist told me that she was retiring at the end of the year. If you can't tell by now, I've had very good relationships with most of my doctors, but few have I been with over 20 years. My dermatologist was one of those doctors.

As you know, I love when a 20-minute doctor's visit feels like a whole therapy session. I like when I am fully heard and seen. My dermatologist was an award-winning doctor who cared. She used to have an office 10 minutes from my home before joining NYU on Wall Street, where I promptly followed. She knew all the doctors in my area and was able to recommend doctors in my network for me to see. She even helped me find another dermatologist to perform a cosmetic procedure because it would be too costly for me at her practice. And when she learned of my cancer, she was a pillar of support. She even ran certain blood work for me when my primary doctor had told me I didn't need it, not even knowing what to do with the results. I adored her so much; her retirement was an excruciating blow.

I wasn't too pressed about finding another dermatologist. Soon after that loss, I received two letters in the mail: one from my insurance company, the other from the Bronx Center. They hadn't come to an agreement, and my insurance was no longer accepted at the Bronx Center. Talk about cutting ties! I understand contract negotiations, but was this legal?

I felt as if minorities in the Bronx were being punished. I wanted to write a letter to everyone about it but didn't have the strength. I was being seen at CTCA, who handled most all of my questions. Occasionally, they referred me back to my primary. It was baffling how a system where all of my medical records were stored for 25 years no longer accepted my insurance.

Even though I was going to CTCA, I still ran to the Bronx Center for quick checkups, urgent care and to see my GYN, Dr. Fabulous. I'd gotten rid of the primary physician who had constantly denied me the tests I needed; I called her *Dr. No.* I got tired of her refusing me! Of course, she's a doctor, and I'm not, but she could've done a much better job. She just didn't want to. Perhaps if *Dr. No* had taken the time to explain why she felt certain tests were unnecessary or that she wouldn't know what to do with the results, I would've been more comfortable with her. She was just so nonchalant about my care! That's why she didn't stay on my medical team for long.

Losing access to my gynecologist was another devastating blow. Akin to my dermatologist, she was another doctor whom I'd seen for over 20 years. Had it not been for her attentiveness, I may never have known I had cancer. She also gave me some of the best life-saving advice in many situations. I'm sure I wasn't the only patient she cared for in a special way, but when she returned my calls on Friday afternoons I felt like I was the only one on her caseload.

Before Dr. Fabulous, I never understood people who used their gynecologist as their primary doctor; however, that's what she became to me throughout the years. For the last few years, my gynecologist acted in that capacity, and I was comfortable with her. I even listed her as my primary on the paperwork I submitted to CTCA.

I brushed my concerns and the pressure to replace my primary and gynecologist aside while CTCA continued taking tremendous care of me. I had no worries...that was until, at the end of 2020, I received the letter stating that CTCA Philly's doors were closing. I was sent into a tailspin. I can't begin to explain how awful I felt; their walls were closing, mine were closing in on me. It was all way too much for me to handle.

ENDINGS - PART 2

~~~

Once the dust settled and the reality of losing my beloved CTCA set in, I was dumbfounded. My first thought was that maybe I could fly to Georgia or Illinois for my doctor's visits. By now, the introduction of COVID was thrown in the mix, making me leery of traveling. But I was willing to do what I needed to do. However, I told myself that as a patient under surveillance and not active treatment, it wasn't a risk worth taking.

To be a surveillance patient is a good thing because you're being monitored annually. This is a positive point of your journey when nothing is going on more than checkups. It's the place of nirvana patients strive for.

I was so connected to CTCA that I was temporarily willing to harm myself by rejecting treatment elsewhere. Changing that one element in my journey changed the entire dynamic. *Be careful what you wish for* wagged its accusatory finger in my face. I'd have to be worse off than I was to still be seen, so I couldn't be mad that my journey with CTCA was ending. I was so devastated I raised the subject often during therapy sessions. Eventually, I came to understand why this was a good thing, but had to deal with the turmoil before I reached that point.

Even though I'd known this was coming for months, I wasn't ready when my final CTCA appointment popped up in June 2021. My doctors kept asking who they should forward my records to, and I had no one. In six months, I'd done nothing to prepare for the end. I wound up taking my scans home, and the rest of my charts were mailed to me.

Not coincidentally, my last appointment with CTCA was an overnight stay, leading into the very last day that the center was open. I usually stayed at the hotel a few miles away, but this was it. I had to stay at the center. It had all the amenities of a hotel, except the floor wasn't carpeted, and it was a tad more sterile. I had stayed there once before for an uncomfortable sleep study with wires connected to me. My last night there was just as uncomfortable. The staff was minimal, it was freezing, and there weren't enough blankets or staff to complain to about it. I mean, the place was shutting down the next day!

I knew CTCA was closing, but on my last day there, I was the very last patient seen by my medical oncologist, breast surgeon, and radiation oncologist. This was now all surreal. It's nothing that I planned, but it was a magnificent last day! As I was leaving, the doors were literally and figuratively closing behind me. I walked out with some of the goods that they were giving away to staff. I have one of the coveted Cancer Treatment Centers of America blankets, and I treasure it. I also received a measuring cup and a few gold starfish, accompanied by a card chronicling CTCA's history.

By the time CTCA shut down, part of my dream team had already moved on to other jobs; the other portion was either undecided or taking time off until they'd determined what their next steps would be. This was huge–the closest CTCA was hours, miles, and states away. With my team scattering everywhere but New York, I was left with separation anxiety, not to mention the added pressure of finding a suitable team to take the old one's place. The mere thought of tackling it alone was daunting. I'd been to networks in NYC but wasn't happy. I'd never be able to recreate what I had at CTCA; I set the arduous task aside for a while.

I put off assembling a new care team for far too long, and procrastination, among other things, started to affect me in late 2021. The impact caused me to have a nervous breakdown–two weeks of not eating, sleeping, or leaving my house. It wasn't just the closing of a center; there were final nails being closed on multiple coffins. My mind couldn't handle all of the immense changes I'd experienced in the last few years.

Even in my distress, I stepped back to look at the bright side. It was time to start everything new. In 2021, I turned 45. Crossing that line was a huge feat for me, as a mere five years prior, I was fighting to live! Now everything around me was dying off, but the atmosphere surrounding me was saying it was time to thrive…and to write.

Remember all those notes I'd taken throughout my cancer journey? I never put pen to paper to actually write the book until the journey was basically over. Writing about my cancer journey was frightening. How dare I move on and live and have the audacity to write about it like it was over? What if it came back? And who made me the authority on this? I called my therapist to get these doubts swirling through my mind worked out. Then, the writing process began.

So many things ending at once broke my heart. But I was also happy for the new beginnings that were flourishing. Cancer gave me character and focus; now it was ending. I was almost lost on what to do next. When you face mortality and come through okay, it's hard to jump to what's next. My desire to live was at an all-time high. I'd gotten so much of what I wanted, but I lacked focus on life after cancer.

Somewhere along the way, I caught a glimpse that it was alright for me to move forward. In order for new things to begin, some things have to end. Make room for the new when you release the old. Like many others, I like to start every new year fresh. Birthdays are like new years to me, but I've actually started living cyclically. From new moon to new moon, every day that God allows us to wake up is a fresh, new start.

SURVIVORSHIP

~~~

At some point, life has to become *MEincorporated.com*. I frequently joked with a sorority sister about having a whole board of directors; however, I was only 75% owner of my own life.

Throughout the journey, doctors tell you what to do next and how to maintain. Then the appointments begin to dwindle, and you start feeling alone and insignificant. While in active treatment, I had an open line to call just about anyone at any time of the day, including a midnight call line to inquire about symptoms I was experiencing. Eventually, it all goes away.

To me, survivorship is what happens after you've completed treatments and you're not under strict doctor's care. Some hate to be called *Survivors*; they prefer *Thrivers* instead. The way I see it, first, you're a survivor, then you're thriving. I am a survivor, and I am thriving! My epiphany came in early 2018. I'd been calling and emailing the doctor's office so frequently about everything, they told me it was time to see

Dr. Percy, who was a joyful survivor himself. Dr. Percy spoke softly and slowly; as a survivor, he spoke from experience that degrees couldn't express.

Dr. Percy was a wealth of knowledge. From our very first conversation, he put me at ease. He also had an answer to all of my questions. What to eat, what supplements to take, how much exercise I needed, and general dos and don'ts. I still recall the sage advice that my breast surgeon once gave me, which is a good reminder for life in general: *If you want to do it and it does not hurt, do it...if it hurts, don't do it.*

My biggest concern about not having constant scans and monitoring was how would I know if the cancer came back or metastasized? There's really no way; however, there are signs to look out for. For example, we should be mindful of losing weight we're not trying to lose, lingering headaches that don't go away, sudden chronic coughing, and unbearable chest pain that wakes you up. Like the start of my journey, I was to schedule and keep up with annual appointments and comprehensive cancer screenings. I also had to adhere to specific guidelines, such as exercising at least 150 minutes per week and keeping my drinking to a minimum or not at all. I'm a social drinker, but I'm cognizant of my alcohol intake since it increases the risk of recurrence.

Since cancer weakened my immune system, my doctor also suggested that I get a multitude of vaccines and medications, including a multivitamin, 80 mg of aspirin, Vitamin D, and melatonin for its immune system properties. He also wanted me to consume less processed foods and consider following a Mediterranean diet.

After my visit with Dr. Percy, I felt equipped to care for myself in the best possible way; I owned my health. Being given a set of rules to govern my steps is how I work best. Dr. Percy positioned me to put my mind at ease. Worrying about everything wasn't helping and made it impossible to live.

Although I've grown stronger, there were still times I got nervous. Like on a business trip to Florida in 2018, when I'd taken a flu shot and my first Prevnar shot. I felt sick; an odd sensation struck that provoked me to call Dr. Percy. Unfortunately, he was busy, so I emailed him with the back story so he'd be apprised of the situation before we spoke. He got right back to me and talked me through a few things to monitor. Admittedly, I was needy and was using my doctor as a crutch. But in an hour of nerve-racking uncertainty, I needed the reassurance.

I must warn you, eventually the team of doctors treating you for cancer goes away. In my case, the center closing is how I lost mine. However, even while CTCA was still open, my visits became shorter, with fewer days on-site and fewer appointments in between general doctor consultations.

These days, I've gone from seeing my cancer treatment team upwards of three times a week to seeing my doctors annually while under surveillance. I was able to start seeing a well-known doctor at Weill Cornell Medicine for a mammogram, MRI, and breast ultrasound as part of my care plan. Keep in mind that for overall health, you still have to see your primary care physician, gynecologist, dermatologist, and dentist–all of the front-line doctors to help with prevention. I've included my long-term naturopath to my complete care team.

Survivorship is the path forward. Just like life, it's a maze of uncharted paths; however, it shouldn't be feared. You have overcome many obstacles to reach survivor status. You've earned it. You're *that* chick. So after all the doctors go away, continue being that chick.

One of the biggest pieces of advice I can give you is to join a long-term support group. Understandably, many survivors want to move far away from anything cancer-related. They don't want to talk or think about what they've overcome, and that's okay. I was the same for a short time. Once we're in remission, why look back? I suppose there's also the nagging doubt of whether cancer ever really goes away. There's always something in my body that goes bump in the night, making me wonder if I'm going to have to go through hell again.

Support groups help take away loneliness and isolation. Our brains love playing tricks on us, making us believe we're the only ones having trouble. When I was first diagnosed, I felt as if no one in the world had ever been diagnosed with cancer before. And with my main support team eventually disbanded, I wondered if I was the only one experiencing this. *This* can be a multitude of adversities. As you open up to more people about your journey, there are a few things that happen, one being people tend to open up about their own struggles, and you realize you're not alone. They may also have valuable resources for you and vice-versa. Accept the gems you are given, and learn from them. Remember, you are not alone; there are others on a journey as well.

JOIN CLINICAL TRIALS

~~~

As per *clinicaltrials.gov*, a clinical study involves research using human volunteers (also called participants) that is intended to increase medical knowledge. There are two main types of clinical studies: clinical trials (also called interventional studies) and observational studies.

While I joined clinical trials throughout my journey and received what I consider life-saving advice and care, I started out as a skeptic. All of this was new to me, and I was terrified. Knowing that my people have been used, abused, and traumatized during studies and trials was frightening. Much has been done to us without permission; however, I was assured that medicine and guidelines had changed, partially due to the patient bill of rights and a study bill of rights.

One thing to note is these clinical trials and studies that I was looking into were not lining up one single group of people. They wanted people of all shapes, sizes, races, and origins. The commonality between us was either breast cancer or triple-negative breast cancer (TNBC).

I took my time, weighing who was doing the study, who was keeping the data, what was being done with the data, and who would be privy to the results of said study, as well as the trial data. I'm big on data security and privacy, and it was hard for me to fathom that I couldn't access my own results. At least I knew my information was secure because almost everything was randomized and by number.

After a while, I just went along with most things presented to me because, at some point, I got the revelation that I was helping more than just myself, like what the cells of Henrietta Lacks did to advance the field of science and medicine. During my five-year journey, I kept hearing medicine has advanced so much since then, all due to research.

My clinical trials began with my genetic testing, which I took through a Bronx network to help decide whether to have a lumpectomy or a double mastectomy. My DNA was tested to determine gene mutations; in my case, if I had the BRCA1 or BRCA2 gene. Luckily, I was negative for both, so I had a lumpectomy. While being seen at the Manhattan Center, I joined a study to dive deeper into my genetics. Ultimately, it was revealed that my cells had a TP53 mutation. The mutation was noted, but it wasn't a huge factor in my treatment plan. Another reason why it's important to join trials and studies when asked; the course of your therapy can change based on what is revealed in a trial or a study.

Because of my survey responses, I was offered to join a trial on the effects of Battlefield Acupuncture. The study involved a doctor checking my pain levels before and after acupuncture. She recorded my levels, then administered acupuncture around my ear lobes. After that, we walked the halls, followed by another pain level gauge. To this day, I'm not sure what made me feel better–the actual acupuncture or the level of care and communication the practitioner extended to me.

What I recall most being in the studies is being evaluated by multiple doctors who aren't just interested in the data. For the most part, I've found those doctors do care about their patient's well-being. During my care and treatment, I never felt rushed. I felt heard and cared for. For the hour I spent with this doctor, I focused on my feelings and pain levels and always left feeling better. As is the case with most studies or trials that I've been in, I never got the results. That is how it usually goes. These studies take time, months, and usually years with hundreds of people. Truthfully, I was bummed at the end of acupuncture because it works, and I was getting it free of charge.

I participated in another study which only required filling out documents and responding to researchers for their studies or thesis papers. I wasn't paid much for any studies or trials, but I did receive random gift cards and Metrocards in the mail for completing them.

There was one study that required daily exercise at the Manhattan Center, but I had to turn it down. As good as the thought of exercise was to me, I couldn't put myself through the wear and tear. Getting to Manhattan on a regular day is a pain, so as a cancer patient with no assistance, it was a solid no. Getting there every day would be too stressful. Now if they had paid for an Uber to get me there and back, I would've been all in. Keep in mind you're allowed to make suggestions that they can agree or disagree to; however, it's up to you to know your body and your limits–do what makes you comfortable and what works for you.

Pearl of Wisdom #19: Before jumping into trials, I suggest you do your research. Thoroughly read the paperwork from start to finish, and consult with your doctor if your decision is impacted by medication. I'm not an advocate of scouring the internet, but you may want to take what other participants are saying into consideration before diving in, too. Gather all the information you need to make an informed decision. As for me, I am a proponent of joining trials.

COOKIE MONSTER

~~~

It's true; idle minds are the devil's playground.

One day, one of my good friends offered me a perfectly legal marijuana cookie with no instructions. It was random; I hadn't been complaining about much, so I assumed she wanted me to have a nice night and relax for a change. On a random Saturday night with nothing to do, I took a bite. Nothing happened. So, I took another bite. After a while, still nothing. Enough with waiting; I ate the whole cookie! Yes, the entire thing. That probably wasn't the smartest thing to do. I called the person to ask what was happening to me and was the cookie good? She confirmed it was fine and told me to relax.

Hours later, I was on cloud 10, past number nine. I was jittery, nervous, and scared. Weed usually causes *the munchies*, but I wasn't hungry. I called Donna, who called my brother Kerry from California. I told them both that I was going to call the ambulance and go to the hospital. Annoyed, Kerry hung up on me.

Donna put me on the phone with a friend whose husband experienced the same thing. They all got a kick out of what was happening! I wasn't angry but glad this was semi-normal, and no one else except me seemed to be worried.

A few minutes later, Kerry called back and told me to relax. "Enjoy the high and go to sleep," he said. Fine, except my body wasn't having that. Sleep wasn't about to happen; he called our cousin who lived nearby. My cousin came to babysit me, pissed that I ate the whole thing without leaving any for her. She had me take a cold shower, then sat with me until I calmed down. She left, and I was asleep an hour later. It wasn't even good sleep. After letting me down, I swore off all things marijuana from that point on.

Because of the hallucinations, hyper anxiety, and speaking truths that needed not to be dredged up, my cousin still calls me the cookie monster to this day. My only other experience with ganja was way back in 1998 in Jamaica. Two puffs and I was clowning. I do remember enjoying myself, though. That night, I sang my best karaoke; that feeling was a stark contrast to this experience.

You may notice throughout this section that I interchange terms often. Over the course of time, I've known CBD to be weed, marijuana, ganja (as spoken by Rastafarians in Jamaica), and Cannabis. Of course, they aren't the same thing, but in my head, they are. It all depends on how it's grown and where you get it. There are different strains and different plants; I typically focus on the strains. For example, indicia is sedating (relaxing), while sativa is energizing. Then there are hybrids, which are a mix of the two. Then there's the little fact of where you get it–the gas station, the weed supplier on the corner, or a sterilized medical facility where it's clinically treated, leaving all the fun out. At least you get the health benefits out of it.

Since the cookie experience, weed was not something I thought about or wanted more of. However, part of my battle with my therapist at CTCA was my not wanting to start anti-anxiety medications. She asked that I consider CBD as an option. Just like the pills she wanted me to take, I was extremely skeptical, but I read how it helped with pain management, potentially minimizing breast cancer recurrence and aiding with overall sleep. Getting adequate sleep alone was more than enough reason to give medical marijuana a try.

Within a few short months, I was authorized to take medical marijuana. When I go to the dispensaries, I'm always sure to refuse *Tetrahydrocannabinol* (THC), the main mind-altering ingredient found in the cannabis plant, which produces the high. I don't ever want a recreational high like my weed cookie night. I just want the medicinal benefits, rest, and calm.

I recently spoke with one of my doctors, who schooled me on the science behind medical CBD. She told me that I was part of a group of pioneers for NYC in 2017 when I was one of the first to get a medical marijuana card and didn't abuse it.

I prefer not to smoke, so before the gummies, I liked the tincture. I added a drop to my tea to relax me and help me sleep. For quicker results, you can place a drop beneath your tongue so it gets into your bloodstream quicker. Still, this wasn't the fastest way to reduce pain, but I'd take it over the effects smoking had on me.

Also, in 2017, there weren't many dispensaries in NYC. I was going to one in Hunts Point in the Bronx, which turned out to be a particularly scary place. The dispensary was nondescript, vanilla, and clinical. They wouldn't let me in until the guard with a gun was present. I also had to show proof documenting my medical issue to gain entry.

Following my first solo visit and purchase, the armed guard asked where I was parked and offered to walk me to my car. Once we got there, I hurried and hopped inside, locked the doors, and raced from the area, vowing never to go there alone again. It's so very different now. The shops are located on the main streets; valid proof is still required to gain entry, but the vibe is totally different.

I still have the hardest time sleeping for many reasons–cancer being low on the list. I don't want my body to ever depend on a specific medication to function. Consequently, I sometimes take CBD, ashwagandha, melatonin with l-theanine, or Tylenol PM. With so many options, it's best to consult with your team to determine what's best for you. By doing this with my own team of doctors, everyone was abreast of the whole picture. And I am happy to say that the cookie monster never reared its ugly head again!

PROCEDURE PREPARATIONS

You will be going in and out of doctors' offices and having many procedures done, getting undressed and dressed multiple times. I didn't have special socks or undergarments but wore comfortable, easy to remove undergarments and clothes so I wouldn't feel rushed or insecure.

Aside from my business suit, on my inaugural visit to my first medical oncologist, I always felt presentable in my black leggings. In addition to that, I wore a camisole with a shirt draped over it to keep the doctors from seeing my breasts. When you're giving blood, they need access to your arm. So that you do not have to strip down to your bra, I suggest wearing a camisole.

Pearl of Wisdom #20: For most procedures like mammograms, sonograms, and MRIs, you should avoid wearing deodorants, lotions, perfume, or jewelry. I'm a nervous test taker, so I carried a stress ball with me to squeeze in my hand. And be sure to know what music you like in the event they ask when testing.

It was during my first MRI that I discovered that I was claustrophobic. A procedure that should take 20-25 minutes took me over an hour. The tech had to pull me out of the machine a few times. I felt so bad for the tech and my friend, who was waiting patiently for me to finish. Make sure to arrive to your appointment early to keep from being stressed out the gate. Bring a relaxing activity to do while you wait, like journaling, a book to read, or coloring. CTCA had these items; however, I wasn't mentally prepared for my first MRI to remember. A few years later, I faced my second MRI. Still terrified, but I went in with a different mindset… and a gummy to keep me relaxed.

As you prepare for surgery, be sure to ask your doctor or the nurse what you can and cannot eat and what medications you're allowed to take. Some medications need to be stopped days in advance of your surgery.

WHAT I KNOW FOR SURE: BONUS PEARLS

~~~

I'm not a doctor; however, there are a few things I'm certain can help you along this journey.

1. Get support, and where possible, surround yourself with supportive people. Support can be in the form of family, friends, and a support group of other survivors. I joined Sister's Network, which is the oldest African-American breast cancer survivorship group in the U.S.

2. Try to minimize or stop drinking and smoking.

3. Exercise when possible, even when the movement is minimal.

4. Adopt a plant-based diet or Mediterranean culinary lifestyle.

5. Do what it takes to manage and control your stress levels.

   • Therapy & Meditation

   • Yoga, swimming, exercise, biking, spa days, reading, or watching funny movies.

6. Take time for you; fill your cup before looking to fill those of others.

7. Don't over-medicate or self-medicate.

   • I advise telling your oncologist and naturopath (if applicable) everything.

8. Ask your doctors' opinions on multivitamins, including Vitamins C and D.

9. Get adequate sleep, even when it's difficult. You must try to rest your brain and restore yourself. To combat this, I suggest melatonin or cannabis. We don't need much melatonin, maximum 5mg, because too much has the adverse effect.

10. Consistently take all of your prescription medications.

11. Maintain or get to a manageable, healthy weight.

12. Use sunscreen.

13. To help prevent lymphedema:

- Fly wearing your compression sleeve.

- Don't get needles or blood pressure taken from the arm that you've had nodes removed from.

HOW I MADE IT THROUGH

∿

God carried me through all of this, but there are some additional things that helped me through.

1. Prayer.

   - Many scriptures in the Bible can be referenced for every situation we face. One that stuck out for me was Ephesians 3:16-21. I learned that by the grace of God, whatever I needed was within me. I went to sleep knowing that God was at work and could shift any storm in my life.

   - Additionally, my college roommate's mother sent me a prayer that I still repeat: *Lord, I thank You for my good health. Heal my body; I know I am well. Let Your will be done in my life. Organize my day and order my steps today and always. Thank You, Lord, because by Your stripes, I am healed.*

2. Going to church.

   - I didn't start going to church when I was diagnosed, I was a faithful member and usher in my church, and my church family was a huge part of my journey.

3. Family time.

   - From beginning to end, my family was a pillar of my strength. That's why I took the selling of the house and my immediate family's move so hard. Having us scattered scared me. But I soon learned that I simply had to love on my family and allow them to love on me. No distance could limit our love for one another.

4. Hanging with friends.

   - Be social, hang out, and enjoy the fun times. I enjoyed fun social gatherings; it doesn't have to be out at a large event. Two or three gathered at your home is great, too. Maybe play games or watch movies. I loved watching romantic comedies and chatting about fun things. No more scary or sad movies for me.

5. Working out.

- Exercise is life; continued movement is a must. I struggle to fit it in now, but it's what keeps the body healthy. Fitness must be a daily part of your life. You can start with the basics of yoga; you don't have to lift weights. Meditation also helps. It may not seem like a form of exercise; however, it helps with deep breathing. Breathwork is needed while exercising. For example, I exhale as I lift and inhale as I lower.

6. Working.

   - This may not be a strong point for most, but work helped me focus on something else besides dealing with cancer. My manager and my team were amazing! Sharing the load helped me see my worth at the company.

7. Listening to my body. Hanging out, working out, and working may not be for you. Do what feels right for you. And at all cost, reducing stress produces positivity that runs through your body.

8. Other activities that I got into:

- I journaled, read more books, colored, and I made tons of waist beads. These activities are all forms of therapy, bringing your mind to a parasympathetic state. They also allow you to release suppressed emotions–remember, suppressing emotions is detrimental to your mental and physical health.

9. Having the desire to live. My desire to live and not give up is a mind-body frequency; there was a love for life, and I wanted to live it. What your mind can conceive, you will achieve.

10. Radically change your diet.

- I'm not speaking of *dieting*—I don't believe in fad diets, but I do believe in eating a healthier diet. I learned from my doctors that a plant-based diet is good for you. Plant-based, no dairy, no red meat, and eating organic can all promote a healthier you.

11. Celebrate your birthdays, successes, failures, and big and small wins.

12. Forgive yourself and others.

A personal development program called *Momentum* helped me find myself. Through this program, I was able to deal with past traumas, which allowed me to forgive myself and others. Additionally, I was able to work on self-improvement and hone my leadership skills.

The American Cancer Society at one time had a slogan titled, *More Birthdays*. Years before I was ever a part of any cancer journey, I was living my best life and taking off for my birthday with more elaborate celebrations than I'd ever done in the past. I'm glad that I started the tradition before cancer; it gave me a sense of purpose and something to look forward to as opposed to doing it because I had cancer.

You can survive through cancer! You can thrive, live, and find joy. Whatever you do for yourself doesn't have to be big and extravagant, either. In 2017, I probably did too much, but it was on par with what I'd done and who I've always been. Because I was in the midst of treatment, I couldn't plan a tropical vacation the way I did in the previous two years. For my birthday, I wanted to be a tourist in my city. I planned a brunch, dinner, and drinks and danced all over Manhattan. I also stayed at a hotel in the city and went to Tiffany's the next day, and made my first purchase there. Celebrating life isn't a catchphrase for me. As long as you have air in your lungs, celebrate in some way.

People may frown upon you doting on yourself, even suggesting you're doing too much, but that's their problem, not yours. Your job is to remain happy, healthy, whole, and complete. Help others along the way, but keep your own cup filled first. It's not selfish; it's life-preserving. Your life. Live for today, always see tomorrow, and know that it's there if you want it and work for it. It's important to keep celebrating life (the good and the bad), have fun, and live!

DO'S AND DON'TS WHEN DEALING WITH CANCER PATIENTS

~~~

Dealing with cancer, whether you're the patient or a caregiver, can be challenging. You don't know what you don't know. It's uncharted territory and a learning experience for all. During my journey, these are some of the things that helped:

1. The main caregivers can push and ask the hard questions.

2. Don't make the cancer patient console you.

3. Be strong, supportive, and optimistic but realistic. It's cancer, and it's serious!

4. Without having gone through it, know that if you are not a doctor in the 21st century, your advice is unsolicited and without medical backing.

5. Don't say, *"Oh, my friend died from ABC."*

6. Do ask if they need help, rides to appointments, or someone to talk to or watch television with. Then actually show up, and follow through on your word.

7. Every conversation doesn't have to be about cancer.

8. Do offer. Articles or advice with searchable sources. Use your best judgment.

9. Don't treat the person as if they are dying tomorrow unless they really are. It's okay to care and support and be gentle. However, while they won't break, use your best judgment or simply ask.

10. No question is dumb, but too much questioning is annoying. Many going through this journey have to repeat the story many times to other friends, family, HR at work or on forms, and even to new doctors. Some write blogs, so you can read about it, and others write books.

11. For the cancer patient–eliminate toxic people and situations while you're in the process of healing. You can't have your body fighting too many toxic situations.

12. I read once, "Would you rather be right or happy?" I choose happy and healthy all the time

I learned that I survived cancer for a reason, and I lived. God's mercy was upon me; the same grace and mercy is upon all of us daily. So don't hesitate to live life to the fullest! Don't settle for anything less than the best because you're worth it.

EPILOGUE

Lena Horne has been quoted as saying, "It's not the load that breaks you down: it's the way you carry it." And I agree, cancer is a heavy load to carry. What I gave you here in the pages of this book are just a few *ways of being* that helped me to move forward fearlessly and with purpose. However, you will determine what is best for your journey.

I choose to reflect on my experience in a positive light because I learned so much. I learned to be vulnerable, to teach others how to love me, and really, in the end, how to love myself better.

Using the *Pearls of Wisdom*, I hope that along your journey, you find the positives that help to keep you pushing forward toward health. I'm rooting for you and am here to support you. So, please visit my website to connect and engage with me and let me know about your journey. And, of course, feel free to share your *Pearls of Wisdom* to support other Thrivers in our online community.

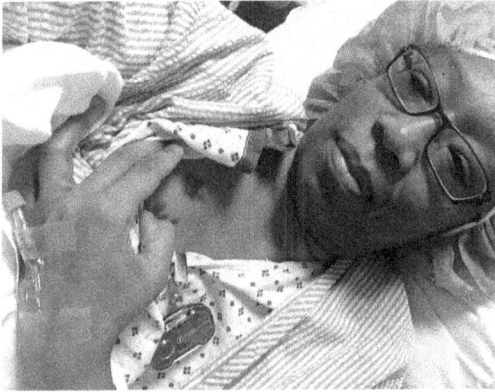

1st Surgery - let's get 'er done (November 2016)

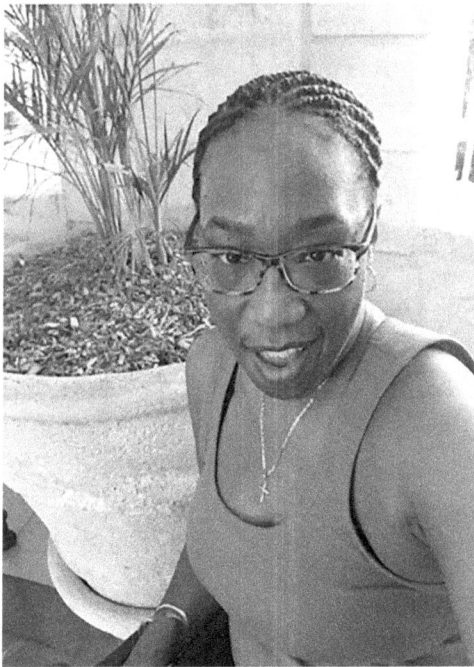

"Ugly Duckling" in Barbados (December 2016)

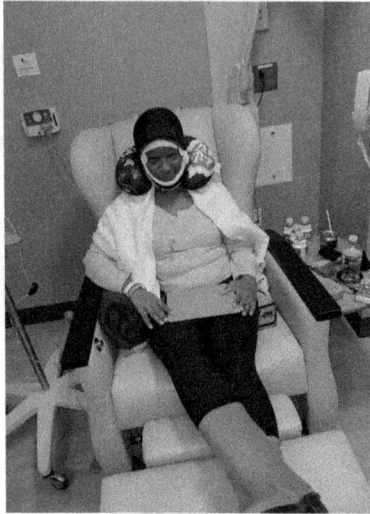

Donning my cold cap during chemo (February 2017)

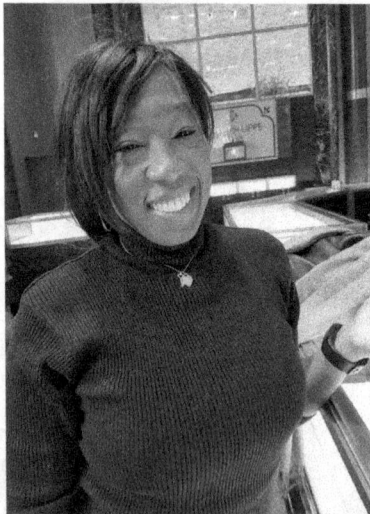

Birthday breakfast at Tiffany's (March 2017)

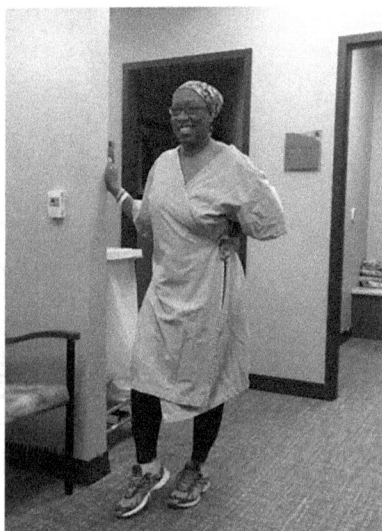

Profiling for my 2nd surgery (May 2017)

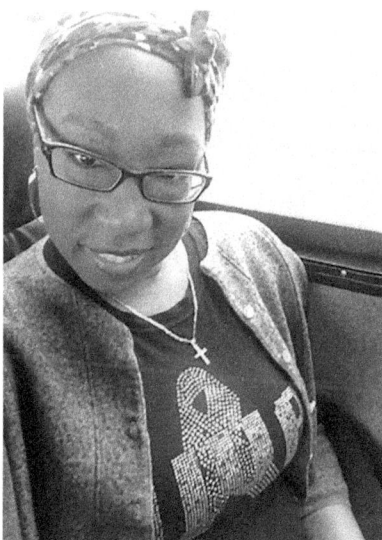

"1st Day of School" bus ride to radiation (June 2017)

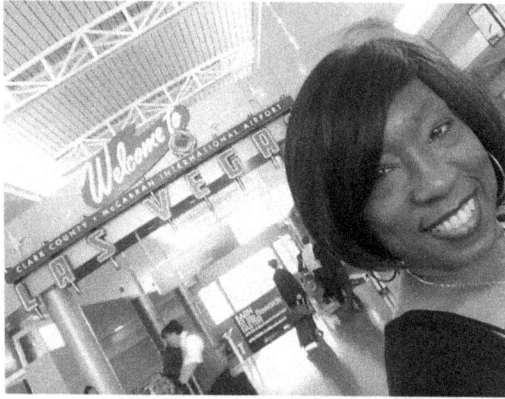

"Hot Head" in Vegas (July 2017)

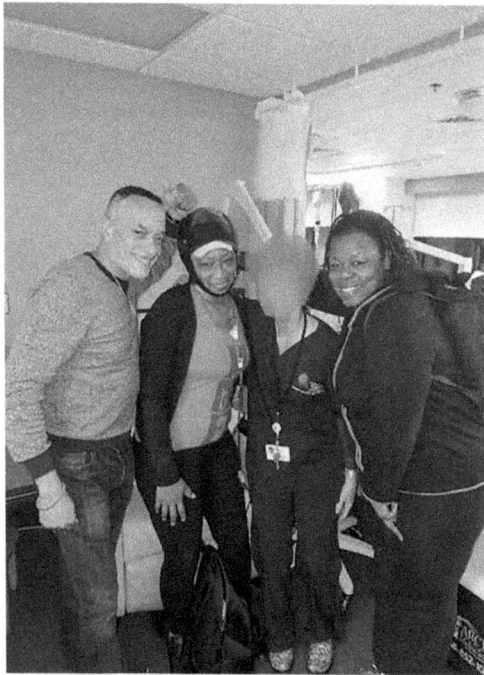

Celebrating my last day of chemo with my caregiver crew

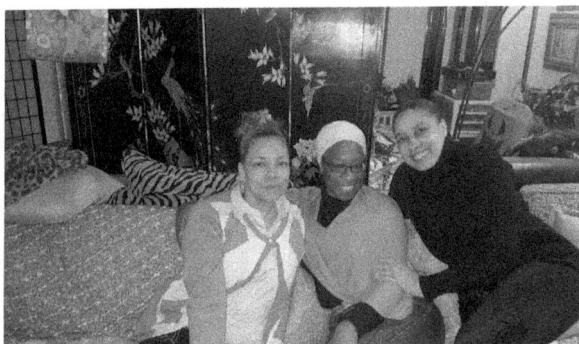

My cute, caregiving sisters

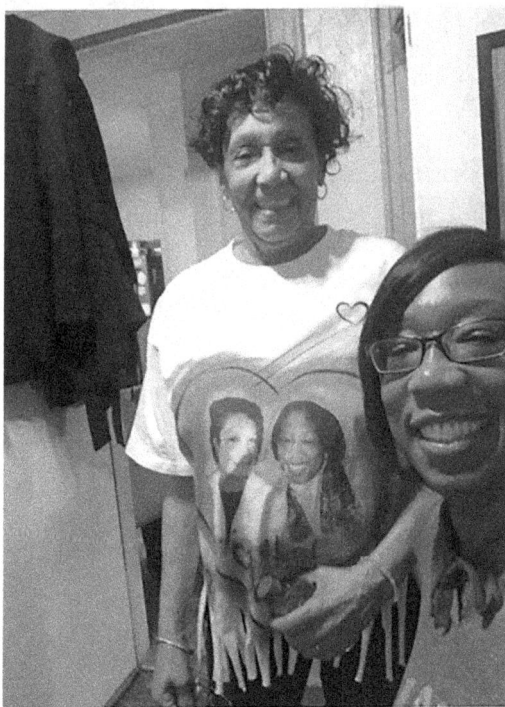

The original caregiver, my Mom

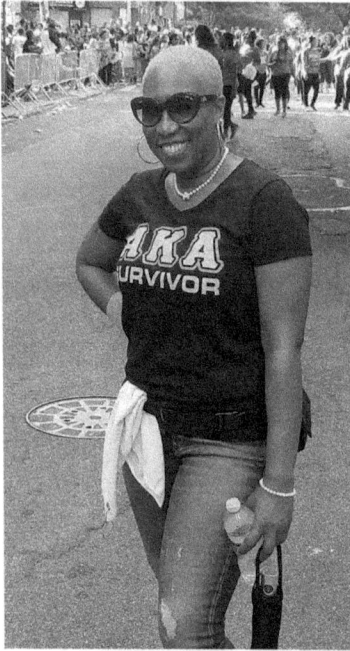

Big Chop
(September 2017)

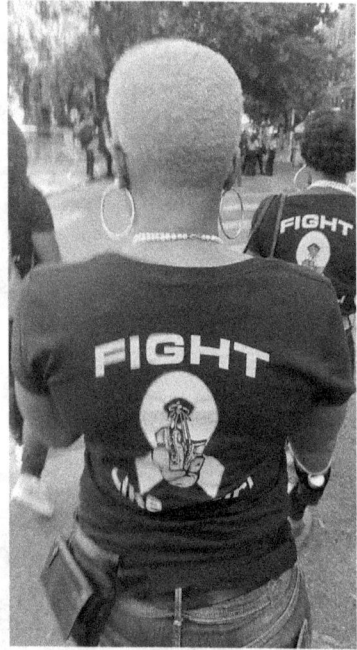

Big Chop - Part 2
(September 2017)

APPENDIX

~~~

Below are a few resources mentioned throughout the book. However, please note that websites constantly change. Check out my site, PINKPOWERSTEPS.COM for additional resources.

CAREGIVERS:

- Healthy Tissue Bank - https://komentissue-bank.iu.edu/about-ktb/our-history.php (Care-givers can help by donating healthy tissue.)

FOOD/FINANCIAL SUPPORT:

- Meals on Wheels - https://www.citymeals.org/
- Needy Meds - needymeds.org (Provides help with cost for medications.)
- Sisters Network Breast Cancer Assistance Program (BCAP) - sistersnetworkinc.org

- WTC Compenstation Fund - https://www.vcf. gov/policy/eligibility-criteria-and-deadlines (Great resource if you believe your cancer was due to being in or near the WTC.)

GENERAL RESOURCES:

- American Cancer Society - https://www.cancer.org/

- Cancer and Careers - https://www.cancerandcareers.org/en (Empowers and educates people with cancer to thrive in their workplace.)

- Cleaning for a Reason - https://cleaningforareason.org/openings-york/

- Clinical Trials (TNBC) - https://clinicaltrials. gov/ct2/show/NCT00532727

- Findhelp.org - www.findhelp.org (Offers a number of services, including legal services.)

- NYC Cancer and Prevention Information - https://www.nyc.gov/site/doh/health/ health-topics/cancer-prevention.page

- Support Group for African-American Women - https://www.sistersnetworkinc.org/

- Triple-Negative Breast Cancer Trials - https:// app.emergingmed.com/tnbcf/home

Hair Care:

- Cold Caps - http://www.rapunzelproject.org/coldcaps.aspx

- Hair to Stay - https://hairtostay.org/

Miscellaneous:

- Ring Theory - https://www.latimes.com/opinion/op-ed/la-xpm-2013-apr-07-la-oe-0407-silk-ring-theory-20130407-story.html

Transportation

- Road to Recovery - https://www.cancer.org/support-programs-and-services/road-to-recovery.html

- Uber - Uberhealth.com

ABOUT THE AUTHOR

Author Tricia Griffith wears many hats; she's a Certified Project Manager, member of *Alpha Kappa Alpha Sorority Incorporated*, Board Member of *Sisters Network*, New York City Chapter, volunteer and community activist. She also holds membership with *The National PanHellenic Council (NPHC)*, *Top Ladies of Distinction* and her alma mater's *Black/Hispanic Alumni Association*; supporting activities in and around her community.

Most notably, she is a breast cancer survivor and advocate. Tricia enjoys volunteering with the *American Cancer Society Cancer Action Network* to improve policies around cancer research, treatment, etc. Volunteerism is important to Tricia and allows her to give back to her community and the causes near and dear to her heart.

In her spare time, Tricia serves as an Usher at her church and loves running (she completed the *Diva Half Marathon*), traveling, event planning, and enjoying a good meal and hearty laughs with family and friends.